SMILE AND JUMP HIGH!

...the true story of overcoming a traumatic brain injury

Donald J. Lloyd and **Shannon L. Kehoe**
With major contributions from
Susan E. Lloyd ❖❖❖ **Kelley A. Lloyd**
Brian D. Lloyd ❖❖❖ **Michael J. Kehoe**

StarLight Press
1090 Overlook Lane
Monroe, Georgia 30656
(770) 266-7791

This Publication is designed to provide accurate and authoritative information in regard
to the subject matter covered. It is sold with the understanding that neither the author
nor the publisher is engaged in rendering legal, accounting or other professional
services. If legal advice or other expert assistance is required, the services of a
competent professional person should be sought.
>   *--From a Declaration of Principles jointly adopted by a Committee*
>   *of the American Bar Association and a Committee of Publishers.*

Library of Congress Control Number: 2001117929
ISBN   0-9673887-2-4

StarLight Press
1090 Overlook Lane
Monroe, Georgia 30656

Maple-Vail Book Manufacturing Group
Post Office Box 2695
York, Pennsylvania 17405

Ordering Information
Telephone orders: (770) 266-7791
Fax orders: (770) 266-7792
Internet orders: **http://www.starlight-group.com/starlightpress.htm**

This book is dedicated to Claud and Mary Catherine Eason;
parents of three, grandparents of seven, and great-
grandparents of three more gifts from God. You have been
the stability and true inner strength for the entire family.
We thank you for the values you have given us, and a
lifetime of love, support and friendship.

TABLE OF CONTENTS

ACKNOWLEDGEMENTS

Barbara Bush clearly had it right when she said, "Cherish your human connections: your relationships with friends and family." In the end, isn't it all that really matters?" Those relationships are what motivated us to write this book.

It is truly impossible to adequately express our heartfelt appreciation for the many contributions made by our family and friends. Nonetheless, we want you to know that your love, support and encouragement during this ordeal will never be forgotten.

To Sue Lloyd: your resolute strength and patience kept us together. Without you, the ending to our story would undoubtedly have been different.

To Kelley Lloyd: you never failed to sacrifice your own needs for the family, and your unwavering faith was an inspiration to us. You are truly our 'Special K'.

To Brian Lloyd: your insight and perspective kept us grounded and fixed on reality.

To our extended family: Richard & Sandra Eason; Rich & Suzanne Eason; Keith & Dixie Eason; Rick & Kim Smith and their boys, Brad and Brandon; Ken & Robin Lloyd; Lorenzo & Merritt Costantini; Brent & Campbell Lloyd; your support, faith and kindness during the difficult times were a great source of strength.

To the many physicians, therapists, counselors, church members and friends: thanks for your skill, prayers, and positive thoughts. They were powerful medicine, and kept us from giving up when the going got tough.

To the members of the Gwinnett County Fire and Emergency Service who provided life-saving care at the scene of the accident, and transported Shannon and Brice to the hospital: our heart felt thanks for your skill and dedication. You should feel a great sense of satisfaction because you saved two lives that early November morning. There are two families who are very grateful.

To the three Berry College students who happened by the scene at the time of the accident, rendered first aid and called the Rescue Squad: your willingness to get involved saved lives. You displayed courage and true compassion, and your parents should take great pride that they taught their children well. You represent what's right with American youth today.

ABOUT THE BOOK

The events and circumstances contained in our story are completely real. We have used actual names, places and locations in many instances, but did substitute fictitious names or places when we felt it was necessary or more appropriate to do so. These substitutions do not alter the essence of the narrative.

It should be noted that while the book has been edited for spelling, grammar, flow and readability, there are some places where the use of language appears awkward or clumsy. We left these idiosyncrasies because they accurately reflect an ongoing deficit of a traumatic brain injury victim, and should help the reader better understand her constant struggle to communicate.

❖❖❖

"Find ecstasy in life; the mere sense of living is joy enough."
                                                    ---**Emily Dickenson**

"Heat is required to forge anything. Every great
accomplishment is the story of a flaming heart."
                                                    ---**Mary Lou Retton**

"The diary taught me that it is in the moments of emotional
crisis that human beings reveal themselves most accurately.
I learned to choose the heightened moments because
they are the moments of revelation."
                                                    ---**Anais Nin**

"Always, always, always, always,
always do what you are afraid to do."
                                                    ---**Ralph Waldo Emerson**

PROLOGUE

Probably the worst fear of every parent is the dreaded telephone call from the police, hospital or family member informing you that your child has been involved in a catastrophic accident. There's a numbing disbelief, instant denial, and then the immediate rationalization that it's *really not that serious*. The mind simply cannot assimilate that kind of emotional shock at the speed of the spoken word.

The surreal becomes real all too quickly, however, when you begin to ask the inevitable questions that flood your mind. Are you sure? When? How bad is it? Was anyone else hurt? How did it happen? Where is she? It's then that the unthinkable takes shape as the facts begin to paint an indisputable picture. Confusion overwhelms you. What do I do now? Will she live? What if she dies? If she does live, will she be disfigured or impaired? How will we pay the medical bills? Will we be able to adequately care for her? If she dies, where will she be buried? What will we do without her? The questions are endless as you try to sort through all the possibilities.

In the next few hours and days, as the pieces of the puzzle begin to fit together, there's hope and despair, disappointment and elation, personal strength and weakness, and finally the reality that, whatever the ultimate outcome, the lives of family and friends will be changed forever. *Life does go on...* but how we see it is invariably different. We are, after all, a product of our experiences, and once we've lived through a personal tragedy, our perspective on life is never the same.

If you're fortunate enough to have your prayers answered, and against all odds she lives, *what then?* There will be a very long period of adjustment and rehabilitation... with an uncertain outcome. Days and nights are fraught with pain, frustration, aggravation, and more worry. Sometimes there seems to be progress, and at other times there's regression. When will it ever end? The answer is possibly *never*. Such is the nature of a closed head traumatic brain injury.

And what about her? How does she feel? How does she cope? Does she have the capacity to understand what has happened? *Her* frustration may be even more acute than yours. If you're extremely lucky, you may learn the answers to these questions as she, indeed, begins to make meaningful progress. As the months go by, you try to establish a normal life pattern, but it becomes apparent that complete recovery may never come.

After a year, she wants to return to her former life; a job in another city, her old college friends and work associates... *she wants to be a normal twenty-something.* You must let go, but your better judgment says she's not ready. She moves away, and you worry constantly. She finds more frustration as she discovers that she's not the same person she used to be. Her friends' priorities have changed. They're establishing careers, getting married, and living in a new world where she simply does not fit. She moves back home. Her disappointment and struggle are heart breaking. There seems to be no end to the anguish... for her and you.

The doctors say that most of the recovery in brain injuries occurs within six months of the trauma. After that, there may be some incremental progress as she settles into her new persona, but major improvement is rare. You watch in dismay as you realize that this once pretty, gregarious, confident, streetwise young woman has trouble dealing with the simplest of problems. Can she hold down a job? Will she ever have friends? Marriage and children seem out of reach. If this is all there is, you ask, would she have been better off to have died that terrible day? Guilt is everywhere. The family feels it and outsiders see it.

Life is truly a mystery... uncertain at best, and as unpredictable as the weather. After a struggle of three years, a friend comes into her life. He didn't know her before the accident. He knows her as she is now, not as who she used to be. As they grow closer, we see drastic improvement in attitude, perception, and her problem-solving skills. We see the emergence of old personality traits. She may not be perfect, but the doctors are clearly mistaken. There's more improvement in year four than in the previous three years combined. They get married forty-six months after the accident. They both have good jobs, and they're happy.

The purpose of this book is three fold. First, it's the chronicle of one brain injury. While every brain reacts differently, each individual experience is important in adding to the limited body of knowledge we have concerning this most mysterious and baffling malady. Secondly, it's a story of one young woman's struggle to regain her life... and her family's torture, hope and elation at a rare success in overcoming the odds. And finally, it's a warning. The entire scenario was preventable. It happened because of a mixture of alcohol and fatigue. Enough said.

Our hope is that this story will give some small measure of hope and comfort to the thousands of families who may unfortunately be forced to deal with brain injuries in the future. Still better yet, we hope that our struggle and suffering will be a lesson to young people and their families everywhere. And maybe, *just maybe*, we can play a positive role in preventing some student or young adult from making a bad choice that results in traumatic injury or death.

---ONE---

The Call

Sunday, November 12, 1995, 6:21 a.m. *Ring... ring... ring...*

"Hello."

"Don, this is Cassie Clark... "

"Oh, my God!"

"Shannon's been in an automobile accident."

"How bad is she hurt?"

"She was on her way back from Athens and lost control of the car. She has some head and chest injuries."

"Where is she?"

"At Gwinnett Medical Center in Lawrenceville. She and Brice were on their way back from the Georgia football game when they ran off the road in a construction area on Highway 316."

"When did it happen? Who was driving? Were they drinking? Why did they call you?"

"It was early, about four-thirty this morning. I'm not sure who was driving, and I don't know whether or not alcohol was involved. Her driver's license has your old Augusta address on it, and they apparently couldn't find your new one, so they called here."

"Cassie, how serious is it? Is Brice hurt? Was anyone else involved?"

"It's serious, but I don't know if it's life threatening. Brice has some injuries, but not as severe as Shannon's. No one else was in the car, and as far as I know, there was no other car involved. You need to call the hospital to find out more. I'm sure you can get the telephone number from Directory Assistance."

"I called her grandmother looking for you, and also tried unsuccessfully to reach Brian. We're leaving for the hospital right now. The hospital representative was pretty concerned, and they want you here as quickly as possible."

1

"We're on our way," I said as I hung up the phone, still half-asleep and dazed with emotion.

I had taken a new job in Murfreesboro, Tennessee in March, 1995, and was living in a small apartment while my wife, Sue, remained in Augusta, Georgia to sell our home. In addition to being the Executive Director of a large medical clinic, I also happened to be serving as the national president of the Medical Group Management Association. Sue had joined me a few days earlier to travel to Chicago, where we had spent time planning our Association's annual convention. We had returned to Murfreesboro late on Saturday night and caught the end of the Georgia-Auburn football game on television.

As I stoically trudged up the stairs to the bedroom, I mused at the irony of the previous day. We awakened to a nice snowstorm in Chicago, which had disrupted the morning airline schedules. We were assured, however, that our early afternoon flight back to Nashville would not be affected. As fate would have it, however, we encountered delay after delay, including a plane without a crew, a crew without a plane, mechanical problems, and finally re-routing on another airline. As the wait at O'Hare Airport stretched into hours, I complained to Sue, *"What else can happen to us?"* Tragically, I found out just a few hours later. I vowed to myself then that I would never again ask that question.

I don't really remember how I broke the news to Sue, but I know she cried. But true to her nature, she quickly composed herself, got on the telephone, and began the task of notifying Shannon's younger sister, Kelley, and older brother, Brian.

It was 6:26 a.m. when the telephone rang at Kelley's apartment. Actually, she was expecting Shannon to call her because they had been playing telephone tag for a couple of days. But the timing was all wrong. After a late night, Kelley was sure that Shannon would not yet be out of bed on a Sunday morning. She sat straight up in bed, but seemed unable to move. The phone rang a couple of more times before Kelley's roommate, Whitney, picked it up. In the blink of an eye she was in Kelley's room.

"Kelley, it's your mother."

"Hello."

"Kelley, it's Mom. Shannon was in a serious car accident coming back from the Georgia game last night. She's in a hospital near Atlanta. Dad and I are leaving right now to go... do you want to go with us?"

"Yes," was all Kelley could muster as a million thoughts gushed through her head.

"Then get on some clothes and get over here now!"

Kelley grabbed her sweatpants, a jacket, a hat and some shoes and raced out the door. It was later that she realized she hadn't showered or packed any additional clothing.

Meanwhile, Sue was on the phone to Brian, who lived in Atlanta. There was no answer, so she left a message on his answering machine.

"Brian... Shannon has been in a very serious automobile accident and is in Gwinnett Medical Center in Lawrenceville. Dad, Kelley and I are on our way. Meet us there as soon as you can."

There was an eerie silence as we brushed our teeth, put on our clothes and quickly packed a suitcase. The quiet was briefly interrupted by a telephone call from Chaplain Marshall of Gwinnett Medical Center. The call lasted less than thirty seconds. Sue was so preoccupied with her own thoughts that she could only recall two things the Chaplain said... *'she's in critical condition, and hurry, but be careful driving'*. In the rush of events, we almost forgot about Haley, our ten year old Border Collie/Springer Spaniel. She had to be taken out and fed, and we had to gather her leash, bowls, food and blanket for the trip.

As I ate a bowl of cereal, my mind wandered, randomly selecting snippets from Shannon's life:

... the middle child of three, *that's always trouble*... I should have had fair warning from the time she was born that she was going to be the 'high maintenance' member of the family... born just as I was discharged from the Air Force, a new job---*and no health insurance*... of course, she had to be in a breech position when Sue went into labor, causing the obstetrician to delay the delivery for several hours to see if she would turn... finally she decided to cooperate after ten hours of labor by turning into the more conventional head first position... her very *entrance* into the world was a clear signal that she was going to command constant attention...

... it didn't take us long to realize that Shannon was going to be an active child---she was a *perpetual motion machine* from the day we brought her home... and, oh yes, her leg braces at six months of age... a congenital misalignment of her legs and feet required that she have special corrective shoes with braces that were connected by a metal bar... we had to keep that contraption on her all night, and as much as possible during the day... this meant that she was largely immobile for several months until her legs and feet were properly aligned... *oh boy, now we knew we were in trouble*... Shannon didn't disappoint us... she cried, wiggled, and finally found a way to lift up her legs---drop them with a crash, and actually move her crib around the room using the centrifugal force generated by her antics... *it was all out warfare for more than six months*... I don't know why Brian didn't just tie her up and stuff a sock in her mouth to shut her up... oh, well, as it turned out, this 'exercise regimen' was helpful to Shannon later in life, as she became a champion gymnast...

... and how about the child gate caper?... when Brian began to crawl, we put him in the back bedroom with some safe toys and put up a two-foot high door gate... it worked beautifully until he was over two years old... *not Shannon*... when she was less than a year old, I put up the gate and lifted her into the room... as I walked away she was in the hall right behind me... I tried again---and watched her climb right over it... I just folded up the gate, never to be used again! ...

...she loves people and lots of activity---and craves approval... she's curious and daring, and has never met a stranger... she has this special charisma that draws people... now she's alone, lying motionless in a strange hospital... fighting for her life! ...

It seems so incongruous.

I was startled out of my trance as Kelley rushed in the back door of the apartment. "Mom, what happened? How bad is she hurt? Can't we..."

"I don't know. The Chaplain called and said it was serious, but that's all he knows. Just get your things into the Jeep and let's get going."

I honestly don't recall what happened after that. I only know that the next time I was aware of time and space, we were on Interstate 24 headed to Atlanta.

---TWO---

The Surreal Trip

7:05 a.m.

We were all lost in thought as we sped down the Interstate toward Atlanta and the unknown. Is it really *that* bad? Sue and I had conflicting opinions. She didn't think so:

... **she'll be okay---she always is... another near disaster... she's tough and we'll find a way to cope while she's recovering... it's just like her broken leg and knee surgery... on her fourteenth birthday, nonetheless---she breaks her leg and jams her knee cap into her thigh on the vault at practice... taken to the hospital in an ambulance... and Don and I rushing to the hospital only to find her 'relaxing' in the emergency room with a bubble cast on her leg...** *she never even cried...* **even that turned out well, as she met her best friend, Jennifer, on the first day of the ninth grade... I'll never forget the story about Jenn tipping Shannon over in her wheelchair... and the football coach carrying Shannon up and down the stairs between the first and second floor...**

As we made our way toward Chattanooga---the halfway point to Atlanta---I began to suspect that this wasn't just another of Shannon's little adventures. I now realized that it was serious. And while I didn't want to allow myself to believe her injuries were really life threatening, I started to consider all of the possibilities, and began to develop a plan for dealing with the details in the event of her death.

It seems odd to me that I never considered any middle ground. I thought she was badly injured, but would heal and fully recover... or she would die. The idea that she might be partially or totally disabled never occurred to me. In contrast to Sue, my thoughts were more ominous:

... if she dies, where will we have the funeral?... who should we bury her?... who will speak for her?... she's so young and has so much more of life to live... I know she would want someone to speak for her... I guess it will have to be me.

Shannon was one of my mother's five grandchildren. And clearly her favorite. It wasn't hard to understand why, since there was a striking physical resemblance, and perhaps an even stronger personality connection. These characteristics were passed from mother to son to daughter---which, of course, made for an interesting relationship between the three of us. Shannon and my mother had the same energy and strong-will, and penchant for finding themselves in difficult situations. Until now, she always seemed to find a way to thrive in the midst of that chaos.

My mother died of emphysema three years earlier, and was buried in Norcross, Georgia under a large oak tree. True to her nature, she had chosen her exact burial site before the cemetery actually opened. Since my stepfather had remarried, it appeared that there would forever be an empty plot next to her. It only made sense that Shannon be buried next to her soul mate.

"Honey, if she dies, we'll have the funeral at the Peachtree Chapel and bury Shannon in the cemetery next to my mother." Sue said nothing, but just looked at me as though I had violated a sacred covenant not to discuss such things. I said no more.

... what is he talking about? ... she isn't going to die... it's not that serious... there he goes again, overreacting without having all the facts... she has some broken bones and was knocked unconscious, but she'll be awake and anxious when we get there... it will be just like a dozen times before--- we'll worry a lot, it will be disruptive, but we'll deal with it...

8

Kelley said nothing. She feared the worst from the time the telephone had awakened her from a deep sleep. At age twenty, the youngest of our children, Kelley is quite special. When she was less than a year old, we discovered that she was hearing impaired---not totally deaf, but with enough deficit that it shaped her personality, social relationships, and view of the world. She spent her formative years undergoing test after test, experimental ear surgery, endless auditory therapy---and learning how to survive in the hearing world.

In a strange way, Kelley's disability worked to her advantage as a person. She learned to enjoy reading---both books and personalities. She developed a strong sense of empathy and a keen insight into the feelings, needs and suffering of others. During those difficult years, Shannon was often her surrogate mother. The bond between these two sisters was quite unique. Now it was her turn to be the caretaker. She both feared and relished that role:

... how could this happen?... Mom and Dad have lectured us a thousand times about being careful while driving... is Dad right?... is she going to die?... I could have stopped it... if I had gone like I was supposed to, *I could have stopped it*... we need her... *she's got to be okay*... Shannon, I love you... please don't die... please don't die... use my strength, *but please don't die*...what am I going to do? ... I won't allow myself to think about that...

Kelley believed she could save Shannon through the power of her thoughts. As she sat pensively in the back seat, the words of the Mary Chapin Carpenter song *This is Love* reverberated in her head:

"...If you ever need to hear a voice in the middle of the night...

when it seems so black outside that you can't remember light...

ever shone on you or the ones you love, in this or another lifetime...

9

and the voice you need to hear is the true and the trusted kind,

With a soft familiar rhythm in these swirling unsure times...

When the waves are lapping in and you're not sure you can swim,

well here's the lifeline... If you ever need to feel a hand, take up your own...

When you least expect, but want it more than you've ever known,

well baby, here's that hand and here's my voice that's calling...

This is love...all it ever was and will be... This is love.

And I see you still and there's this catch in my throat, and I just swallow hard til it leaves me.

There's nothing in this world that can change what we know,

but I know I am here if you ever need me... And this is love..."

In just two hours we passed through Chattanooga and were on Interstate 75 near the North Georgia border town of Ringgold. We were still two agonizing hours away from our destination.

"I'm going to stop at the Exxon station and call the hospital," I said to Sue as I pulled in to get gas.

"Okay, but hurry up. We need to get there as soon as possible."

What followed was the first of many frustrations to come. For some reason, the pay phone wouldn't let me make a long distance call. The Chattanooga operator tried to explain why, but it only increased my irritation. I finally gave up and jumped back in the car.

"I couldn't get through," I muttered to Sue and Kelley. "I'll have to try again a little closer to Atlanta." With that, we were off again.

Dalton, Georgia was the next town, about 20 miles away. I was thinking that I'd stop there to make the call when I saw a sign pointing the way to a Georgia Highway Patrol Station. I quickly turned off and followed the signs less than a mile before I saw the office up a steep hill on the left. I pulled up to the building and it looked abandoned.

There was one civilian car in the parking lot---and absolutely no signs of life. I jumped out and went up to the door. I clearly startled the two young officers on duty, who really didn't know what to think when I rang their doorbell.

"Uh, yes... well, uh... can we help you?"

"I need to use your telephone. My twenty-four year old daughter was in a serious accident in Lawrenceville, and I need to find out her condition."

"Okay, come on in," one officer replied somewhat tentatively. He then buzzed open the security door and let me in.

As is my temperament, when under pressure, I tend to take command. I immediately began barking orders to the officers. "I don't have the number. I need a telephone book. I need to call the fourth floor ICU waiting room at Gwinnett Medical Center. Where's the phone? Do I need to dial 9?"

The two officers scurried around attempting to accommodate my demands. They called Information and quickly obtained the telephone number. Within a couple of minutes, they dialed the number and handed me the telephone.

"Hello, this is the ICU waiting room," came the reply after a couple of rings. The voice was familiar. It was my brother-in law.

"Richard, it's Don. What can you tell me?"

"Where are you?"

"We're just over half way, at the Highway Patrol Station in Dalton."

11

"You need to get here *right now!*" There was grave concern in his voice. Now I knew it was life threatening.

"How bad is it Richard?"

"The doctors are very uneasy. They want you and Sue here as fast as possible."

"Is she still alive?"

"Yes, she's in surgery, but the doctors don't think she's going to survive."

"Richard, I trust your judgment... you make whatever decisions you have to. We'll be there in a couple of hours."

"Okay, but hurry!"

Now everything began moving at warp speed. I thanked the officers for their help and they offered their condolences. I left the building on the run and leaped into the car. Sue and Kelley could see the obvious distress on my face.

"I talked to Richard. It's critical. She's in the operating room now. *She may not survive until we get there.*" Sue and Kelley sat dumbfounded. From that moment on, we were all in shock. Sue later confessed that she finally gave in to the idea that Shannon might not live, but was so upset that she couldn't recall any thoughts the rest of the way to the hospital. Time was of the essence... and I drove like it.

The remainder of the trip was mostly a blur. I was resigned to the fact that Shannon would be gone by the time we arrived, and I spent the time trying to adjust emotionally to the loss of my daughter. With tears streaming down my face, I tried to think about what she might want me to convey to her family and friends at her funeral. I was in a dreamlike emotional state. I grieved for our loss, but was strangely calm.

I wanted to let Shannon talk to her family and peers one final time through me. The next two hours flew by as I was consumed by my thoughts:

...We have lost a vivacious and talented young woman. And it seems natural to ask why? I'm not going to do that---because there is no good answer. Rather, I want to let Shannon talk to you herself. She's not here in body, but she *is* in spirit. I think I knew my daughter as well as anyone, since she had many of my personality traits, and because she often confided in me. I also believe she was giving me her thoughts in the last minutes of her gallant struggle for life.

'I'm sorry I've caused all of you such grief. I never meant to hurt anyone. I was just living the life God gave me, and I never thought I would... I mean, I'm sorry, it just seems like it was all a terrible mistake. I shouldn't have died... I *couldn't* have died---but I did. I had a great family. I loved my parents, my brother and sister, my grandparents, cousins and friends. I enjoyed life. It was an exciting journey from one fun activity to another. I always knew I was the adventurous sort, but I *never* thought I would do anything that would actually take my life. I just didn't think before I acted. Dad always told us that every mistake could be overcome, every problem solved, and everything broken could be fixed or repaired---except if you killed someone or died yourself. I wish I had *really* understood what he meant.

Mom, you're the best. I tested you a lot. You always passed... and you were always there for me whenever I fell down. I'm sorry I hurt you so much! I know you were so much looking forward to me getting married and having children so you could be a grandmother. I'm sorry I failed you.

Brian, you were the perfect brother for me. I was zany and you were always so cool. You never let things bother you like they did me. I worried a bunch about things that just weren't important. You, on the other hand, just blew them off. How did you do that? You were so smart, and I not quite so. I'll miss your guiding hand.

Kelley, you enriched my life. You endured so much when you were little. I learned that you had patience... and I had none. We had such fun, didn't we? I can't tell you how much I enjoyed being a BIG sister to you. Now you've grown up and turned out to be such a bright and beautiful young women. It pains me that I won't be around to see you reap the rewards in life that you deserve.

Dad, I can't express...'

"Don, there's the hospital sign. Turn right at 120." My thoughts were interrupted as Sue brought me back to reality.

We had traveled 270 miles, with two stops, in less than three hours and forty-five minutes. It should have taken four and a half hours with no stops; and I knew the moment of truth was almost here. I thought I was prepared for the worst as I made my way through traffic and into the parking lot of Gwinnett Medical Center. I was wrong. *My heart immediately sank.* Standing on the curb in the parking lot were my brother-in-law, Richard; his wife, Sandra; and Sue's brother-in-law, Rick. We were now certain that Shannon was gone.

---THREE---

The First Agonizing Day

11:44 a.m.

My heart was racing so fast I thought it was going to come out of my chest. I could hardly breathe. The body language of our relatives demonstrated anxiety, not grief, however.

...so she isn't gone yet. There's still a chance...

Once again, I went into my command mode. "I'll let you and Kelley out at the curb, and I'll park the car and get Haley situated," I said hoarsely.

"We'll wait for you," replied Sue.

"No. I'll catch up with you." With that, Richard opened the door and Sue and Kelley got out. I drove to the back of the lot to find a suitable place to park where the dog would be safe and comfortable. While it was November, the days could still be warm in Georgia, and I was worried about leaving Haley in a hot car for an indefinite period of time. I found a nice shady spot; slightly opened the windows to let in some fresh air, filled her bowl with water, and took off across the parking lot on the run.

"How bad is it Richard?"

"It's bad, Sue. We need to get upstairs as quickly as we can."

"You and Sandra take Sue and Kelley to the waiting room, Richard. I'll wait for Don," Rick instructed.

"What happened? What kind of injuries does she have? Have you seen her?"

"We really don't know much, Sue," replied Sandra. "The accident happened about 4:30 this morning, and she has several injuries to her chest, stomach and head. She came out of surgery about an hour ago. We haven't seen her yet."

It only took a minute for them to get to the elevator and up to the fourth floor. As the elevator door opened, Sue immediately saw her mother and father, Claud and Mary Catherine Eason, standing with the hospital Chaplain. In an instant, I got to Rick and he ushered me up to the waiting room.

We were also greeted by Cassie Clark and Martha Burks. Shannon had recently received her Master's Degree in Interior Design from the Savannah College of Art and Design, where she had been a classmate of Cassie's daughter, Lindsey. She was living with Cassie and her housemate temporarily while looking for a permanent job and place to live.

Chaplain Marshall immediately turned his attention to us. He asked the family to gather around, join hands, and bow our heads in prayer. While I know it was important to ask for God's help, I can only remember being anxious to get it over with so I could go to my daughter. When he completed his prayer, I opened my eyes to survey the situation, and noticed that Kelley was now crying. She feared the worst:

...oh, no, I might never see my sister again. I wish it were me in there...

Chaplain Marshall tried to prepare us for the sight we were about to see as he led us through the double doors of the Intensive Care Unit to Shannon's room. No description of her condition could possibly have been adequate. *Shannon was a mess!*

Shannon had decided that she was going to attend the University of Georgia before she entered the first grade. If Daddy was a Bulldog, then it was good enough for her. She loved sports of all kinds, but gymnastics and college football were her favorites---and Georgia football was at the top of the list.

Her elementary and secondary school education was completed in Birmingham, Alabama, where football is a religion. From the time one is born or crosses the border into the State, he or she is required to declare an oath of allegiance to either Alabama or Auburn. She, of course, would have none of that. She was a Bulldog through and through. She liked Alabama well enough---primarily because she had attended gymnastics camp in Tuscaloosa several times, and loved their coaches. But Auburn was another matter. A despicable Georgia rival, barely to be tolerated.

As destiny would have it, her best friend Jennifer went to Auburn. Shannon visited several times during the college years, and developed relationships with many of Jenn's friends. Likewise, Jenn and her college mates traveled to Athens and developed relationships with Shannon's college classmates. Over a five-year period, a tradition of sorts developed. A group of ten or so would always meet in the town where Georgia and Auburn were playing, would socialize, attend the game, and have a party afterward. This particular Saturday in November was no different.

Shannon had two tickets to the game, and had first asked Kelley to come down from Tennessee to go to the game with her. Kelley had other plans and couldn't come. She also called Jenn, who now lived in Atlanta. She was spending the day with her fiancé, Paul, so Shannon finally decided to ask an acquaintance from work, Brice, to go with her.

She got up early, took her daily run, showered, dressed, decorated her car with Georgia paraphernalia, and went to pick up Brice at the Town Center Mall in Marietta. When they got into her Nissan Sentra, it wouldn't start. They decided to take Brice's car, a bigger, more powerful

1987 Mercury Sable. This would turn out to be both instrumental in causing the automobile accident and saving their lives.

The day went pretty much as planned. They met their Auburn and Georgia friends, tailgated on the Georgia campus, and went to the game just before the 7:30 p.m. kickoff; where they harassed each other unmercifully throughout the evening. Georgia lost in a shootout, 37-31.

They left the campus after 11:00 p.m., and hit a few of the nightspots around town before going to the hotel where some of the Auburn gang were staying. One of her Georgia friends invited Shannon and Brice to stay overnight at his apartment, and while she knew it was a good idea, Shannon just wanted to go home. It was now almost 2:00 a.m. on Sunday morning.

Shannon has never been a big drinker, but many of her friends could 'put it away'. As a result of her conditioning from nine years of gymnastics, she also avoided eating unless it was absolutely necessary. As a result, the two beers she drank after the game elevated her blood alcohol level---not excessively high, but high enough. Brice had consumed entirely too much, and Shannon was not comfortable with him driving. She offered to drive, and he immediately went to sleep as they began the eighty-five mile trip back to Marietta.

While we'll never know the full truth about the accident, we pieced together the following scenario based on the police reports and flashbacks from Shannon.

They were on Georgia Highway 316 in Lawrenceville; about thirty miles from home when the accident occurred. They were in an area where a third lane was being constructed, driving at the posted speed limit of 55 MPH. Shannon was growing tired and she yawned and closed her eyes for a few seconds. *A few too long.*

After taking a deep breath, she opened her eyes to find that she was on the left shoulder of the divided highway, and felt the car begin to slide. She wasn't familiar with its size or maneuverability, and overcorrected. The car then went across both lanes to the right, off a two-foot ledge and into the unfinished third lane of road. Looming in front of her was a fifty-foot cliff.

She also saw a large concrete drainage box that had not yet been buried. She had to make a quick choice. Down the bank or into the box? She thinks she chose the box because she was sure they would overturn if they went over the cliff, and she felt that they had a better chance of survival if they stayed upright.

Brice was still asleep and was totally unaware of what was happening. Shannon believes she rotated the steering wheel so the car would hit the box on her side, hopeful of avoiding any injury to her companion.

Shannon's room in the ICU unit was teeming with activity. There were at least three nurses and two doctors, all tending to a monitor, checking vital signs, adjusting her position in the bed---and working feverishly to keep her alive.

She had a total of nineteen probes, wires, tubes, monitors or braces penetrating or attached to her body. The most frightening being the stent in her brain. It was there to monitor intracranial pressure and brain activity. Then there were the bilateral chest tubes, draining the blood from her lungs into bags that hung on each side of the bed. Both of her lungs had been collapsed and contused, preventing her from breathing on her own. Her breathing was being done by a ventilator, with 100% oxygen, at the maximum possible setting of 20 pounds of pressure.

It was clear from the moment Shannon was brought into the emergency room that she had serious abdominal injuries.   After placing the chest tubes, the surgeon performed an exploratory laparotomy and found that her bladder was torn in five places, and its contents had spilled into the abdominal cavity. He had to clean the area and repair the ruptures in her bladder.

Her spleen was also leaking some blood, but not enough to require removal of the organ. The laparotomy incision that ran from just below her breastbone to her pubis had been packed, but left open for drainage. There was a tube protruding from that wound, as well as a catheter from the bladder itself.

Because they didn't know how bad her neck injury was, Shannon was fitted with a cervical collar, which remained in place for the first several days. She had a feeding tube in her nose, which had literally been obliterated at impact, along with her beautiful high cheekbones. The suspected stress fractures to both eye orbits and her left hip were of little concern because they were not life threatening. If she *were* to survive, they could be formidable problems to deal with, however. They were simply not a priority at the time. Nor was the broken jaw or major fracture to her left clavicle; where the seat belt had ripped out a two-inch gap.

There were two IVs in each wrist and arm, just below the elbows, pumping life saving fluids and antibiotics into her body. She was hooked up to an electrocardiograph, oxygen monitor and, of course, a blood pressure cuff.

While I didn't have any formal medical training, I had learned a passable amount of medicine from physicians in my twenty plus years as a medical practice executive. *I probably knew enough to be dangerous.* I looked at Shannon carefully for color, breathing and normal signs of life, and surveyed each monitor, pausing at each one to make an assessment:

...her intracranial pressure is in the normal range---

an excellent sign given the apparent severity of her head injury... the lungs don't look good... there's an awful lot of blood in those bags---especially the left one... pulse is somewhat erratic, but not too excessive at 135-140 beats per minute... respirations are high, but not extreme at 28 per minute... blood pressure not bad at 145/80... temperature is a little low... 96.5 degrees... she's out cold... although she does show signs of a pain response when her skin is scratched...

"Mr. and Mrs. Lloyd, I'm Dr. Carter. I'm a pulmonologist. I'm sorry to have to tell you that things look very bad. *It isn't likely that your daughter will survive because of her lung injuries.* She's not breathing on her own... the ventilator has taken on that task. The trauma she's suffered to her lungs has put her at great risk for Acute Respiratory Distress Syndrome, or ARDS. Essentially, that means that the lungs---which are normally soft and spongy---will begin to harden very quickly, and she will forever lose the ability to breathe. I'm afraid it's only a matter of hours, at best. We've had a very difficult time stabilizing her, and some acute event could occur at any time. I'm sorry. We'll do all we can to make her comfortable."

My immediate thoughts were:
...it's not gonna happen! ... the monitors don't look that bad... they don't know how much of a fighter she is...

Dr. Jerry Carter was in his late 30's, with dark hair and a perpetual five o'clock shadow. He was perhaps five feet seven inches tall, seemingly a nervous sort, and was *all clinical*. At the time, he didn't seem to be very likeable. This was just another tragic case for him, or so it seemed at the time.

Standing with Dr. Carter was a pleasant young woman who identified herself as the Head Nurse in the ICU Unit. "I'm so sorry to have to talk with you about this now, but we need to know if you would consider donating your daughter's vital organs? We'll have to begin making arrangements for the transplant procedures as soon as possible."

Sue was completely dumbstruck. She looked at me with complete horror on her face. We had been in the hospital for perhaps ten minutes, and with Shannon for half that time, and they were declaring our daughter dead... and wanted us to donate her organs!

"We'll be glad to donate organs if she dies, but I wouldn't warm up the OR just yet. *I don't think she's going to die!*"

"Mr. Lloyd, it's a virtual certainty," injected Dr. Carter.

"Dr. Carter, is it *possible* to survive those injuries?"

"Yes, but only one in a hundred could be expected to survive," he replied in his best clinical mode.

"Well, I respect the fact that you know medicine... *but I know the patient!* I'm convinced that she will live." Apparently I responded with such force and conviction that everyone in the room stopped what they were doing and looked at me. Everyone thought I had completely lost my mind except Sue. *She believed.*

With that, Dr. Carter and the nurse scurried off. Sue and I went to the bedside, gently rubbed Shannon's hand, and told her we loved her. I also told her I was giving her all of my energy and strength, and that she had the good thoughts and prayers of her family to rely on.

"Sleep well, sweetheart. You're going to get through this."

It was about eight hours after the accident, and the ICU waiting area was crowded with extended family and friends from the Atlanta area. Brian had arrived, and he and Kelley were somberly talking with family members gathered in the area as they awaited word from us.

As Sue and I walked through the double doors of the ICU, we could see the grief stricken, solemn faces that filled the room. Fear and a sense of inevitability pervaded the air. They had already begun to grieve Shannon's loss.

"It looks very bad," I began. The doctor doesn't expect her to live. *But he's wrong!* I looked at the monitors and I believe she's going to make it. Her lungs are the major problem at the moment, but she's young, healthy and athletic, and I'm convinced that she's going to survive!"

Sue was transfixed as she tried to find some order in the chaos:

...everyone faces a crisis differently... they protect themselves by withdrawing, crying, analyzing, praying---or in Don's case, by *acting*... I don't think he really believes Shannon's going to live... it's just his way of coping with the stress... I don't know what to think... he *does* have some knowledge of medicine... but doesn't the doctor know more? ...*I want to believe him*... is he acting, or does he really believe? ...

Suddenly the room seemed in a roar. Everyone had questions. They wanted to know about each injury. They wanted to know when she might wake up. They wanted to know how long the recovery period would be. Questions that simply couldn't be answered at that moment. Sue and I briefly related all we were told and what we observed. Kelley and Brian wanted to see Shannon.

Because there were other patients in the Intensive Care Unit, and almost complete quiet was essential, only two people were allowed in the Unit at a time. I took Kelley in first, while Sue stayed to answer questions and take the now mounting number of telephone calls.

When Kelley saw her big sister lying in the bed with all the probes and monitors, her heart broke into a thousand pieces. She could hardly believe what she was seeing. She was determined to be strong, however, so she sucked it up and walked over to her side:

23

...she seems almost peaceful... her face is so swollen that it doesn't really even look like her... it's almost as if someone has taken a dummy and made her resemble my sister... *it's not real*... any minute now Shannon will come walking in here and ask us why everybody is crying... she's stubborn... she can handle it... I believe Dad, if he says she's going to make it, with God's help, *she will*...

"Shannon, I'm here. I'll be here for as long as you need me. Whatever it takes."

Brian was next. He was in shock. He was twenty-six years old, and had recently moved to Atlanta after working in Gainesville, Florida for four years following his graduation from the University of Florida. Brian is not a big talker. His IQ is in the top one percent, and he just doesn't usually engage in small talk. He prefers not to waste his words, and when he's ready, he almost always has something meaningful to say. He's also not easily impressed.

I remember once in 1984 when Brian was fourteen years old, he and I were in a mob at Sanford Stadium in Athens where Georgia and Clemson were in the midst of a tense battle late in the fourth quarter. The crowd was almost hysterical, as the Georgia place-kicker, Kevin Butler, lined up to attempt a school record 60-yard field goal to win the game. He looked at me calmly and assured me that Number Five would make it. He did. Brian just smiled and said, "I told you..."

Seeing his sister in a life-threatening situation *impressed* Brian. He, like Sue, had initially thought this was another one of Shannon's semi-serious predicaments. It was clear to him now that her condition was critical. It showed in his face.

Sue spent much of the day by Shannon's side. Kelley and I were in and out of the Unit, talking with well-wishers, taking telephone calls from friends, and meeting with physicians who had already treated Shannon or would participate in her care in the coming days or weeks.

Kelley and I are both pretty verbal when it comes to our feelings, and it helped to be able to vent to each other. Brian stayed in the waiting area for most of the day because he was in the early stages of a cold, and did not want to spread his germs to Shannon. The virus actually forced him to stay away from the hospital for a couple of days later in the week.

By mid-afternoon, the adrenalin rush began to subside, and fatigue set in. We also realized that we hadn't eaten since before 7:00 a.m. We got a Diet Coke and some crackers out of the vending machine, and continued our vigil. At appropriate times, we were able to take some family members back to see Shannon. Each of them was appalled at how bad she looked, and most were startled by all the monitors and tubes. While no one actually said it, to a person, they believed she wouldn't survive. Their body language belied their pretend optimism.

I had not called my stepfather, my brother, or any business colleagues or friends because I wanted time to fully assess the situation before talking with them. By 4:00 p.m., Shannon was stable and didn't seem in imminent danger of a fatal event. There was no change in her breathing, and the chest tubes continued to drain copious amounts of blood. Her pulse rate had declined slightly, and her blood pressure continued to be stable, if a little high. Perhaps more importantly, the electroencephalogram (EEG) showed measurable brain activity and high normal intracranial pressure.

I notified my stepfather, who lived in Woodstock, Georgia, about an hour and a half away; and my brother, Ken, who lived in Houston. Ken offered to catch a plane to Atlanta immediately if we needed help. I asked him to wait a few days until the confusion abated. I called my friend and colleague, Fred Graham, who was the Associate Executive Director of the Medical Group Management Association in Denver. Finally, I called Judy Primm, our Assistant Administrator at the Murfreesboro Medical Clinic.

It was a very difficult series of phone calls because I had to 'relive' the horror of the situation four times. It was necessary, however, because each of these people played significant roles in our lives, and arrangements had to be made to cancel travel plans or meetings during the next week.

Somewhere in the middle of the day, most of the friends who spent the previous day and evening with Shannon in Athens arrived. Some had gone back to Auburn, a couple to South Carolina, and several to their homes in various cities across the state of Georgia. They were stunned and shaken, and simply couldn't believe they were in danger of losing their energetic and steadfast companion.

I quizzed them about what they had done the night before... and if Shannon had been drinking. They swore that she only had two bottles of beer the entire evening--- and, of course, *nothing to eat*. They apologized for not forcing Shannon and Brice to stay in Athens until morning. Like most of us when a crisis occurs, they played the 'if only' game. If only we had forced her to stay. *If only...*

Before the end of the day, there were over fifty visitors. Most stayed until well into the evening. There were also telephone calls from dozens of our friends and colleagues from Alabama and around the country. We were moved by the outpouring of love and encouragement.

A support system is absolutely crucial during times of adversity or distress. Without it, hardship often consumes those in crisis, and the long-term outcome is frequently calamitous. They are formed by a web of friends, family and neighbors who almost seamlessly integrate themselves into the sufferer's daily lives by taking on physical tasks like cooking and cleaning, running errands, and providing time for an occasional escape from the crisis.

More importantly, however, these individuals also become the emotional foundation that keeps order and normalizes perception. They are alternately laborers, caregivers and counselors---and without them, it's easy to lose hope and focus. There is no training for this role, and the only qualifications needed are unexpected circumstances and a willingness to contribute to the well being of others.

In short, the people who comprise the support system bring the balance and perspective that is badly needed during traumatic times.

Over the next few hectic weeks and months, we had an extraordinary group of people who provided our support system. Shannon's grandparents, aunts, uncles and cousins; family friends; colleagues and associates from Alabama and Tennessee; several physician friends; and many others. While each individual in this group played an important role, there were three amazing young people who redefined the word loyalty.

Jennifer Behrens is, like Shannon, one of three children. In her case, the youngest. And an absolute bundle of energy. She is slightly built, but never shy about voicing her opinion on matters, and certainly not one to be bullied or taken advantage of easily. She and Shannon were constant companions during the junior and senior high school years. One might have thought that going to separate colleges would diminish the relationship, but on the contrary, they burned up the telephone lines between Athens and Auburn.

Jenn was a very talented student, particularly in

math, and she literally carried Shannon through her struggles with algebra and trigonometry in high school. Shannon was the admired athlete and social butterfly. Jenn was a second sister to Shannon, and a favorite third daughter to us. She was a tireless caregiver and therapist immediately after the accident and throughout the long recovery period.

Shannon met Samy Iskandar as a freshman at the University of Georgia. They were housed in the same dormitory for two years, and they were friends from the moment they met. Samy is short, perhaps five-foot six, but nobody ever told him. He simply doesn't recognize roadblocks. He also loved UGA life, the football team, and people.

They talked in person or by telephone virtually every day during their four years in school, and almost as often afterward. Samy is seemingly always the optimist, even in the face of adversity. This was very important during the times of uncertainty in November and December.

It's important to note that Samy had wanted to go to medical school since he could remember. He studiously prepared himself at Georgia, and was admitted to the Medical College of South Carolina, near his home, in 1994. Within a few weeks of registration, however, he hurt his knee and had to have surgery. As fate would have it, he had a post-operative infection that threatened his life, and he was unable to begin classes until much later.

Shannon provided support and encouragement to him on a daily basis. Now it was his time to return the favor. He was at her bedside constantly in those first days, providing optimism and much needed levity. This was a major sacrifice, since he was in the middle of med school exam week. As an aside, he is now Dr. Samy Iskandar, Obstetrician/Gynecologist.

The third remarkable friend was Kim Black from

28

Tucker, Georgia. She was Shannon's sorority sister and roommate during the last two years of college. Kim is as pretty as a picture, always has a smile, and possesses an infectious personality. She can charm the honey out of a beehive.

They were also classmates in the Interior Design Program, had similar tastes and talents, and made an energetic pair. Kim provided daily vigil, encouragement, and bursts of self-deprecating humor when our perspective needed to change.

Fatigue and darkness typically has a debilitating effect on one's psyche during a crisis...and as the eventful day moved toward evening, things looked less optimistic.

Early in the day, Dr. Carter had indicated that ARDS would begin to set in about twelve hours after the initial injury, and the critical stage would be the following twenty-four hour period. We were now entering that time, and we increased our awareness of the monitors and chest drains. The slightest change of any kind seemed to signal that a fatal event was rushing toward us.

We held Shannon's hand, talked to her, prayed, and told her how tough she was. We'll never know whether or not this helped, but it was important to us to emit a presence of hope.

Gradually, many of those who spent the day in watchful waiting began to filter away---some to go home to their families, others to get away from the bedlam for awhile, and still others to eat dinner. Kelley, Brian, and I took Haley over to my mother-in-law's house to get her situated, and to have some dinner. We then prepared a plate to take back to Sue at the hospital.

At various times during the day, the nurses or doctors would ask us to leave the ICU so they could examine Shannon, change linen, adjust IVs, or take care of some other housekeeping chore. Around 6:30 p.m., while Sue was sitting alone outside the Unit waiting for the nursing staff to complete their work, a pleasant appearing woman in her late twenties approached her.

"Mrs. Lloyd, my name is Kathy Dunbar. I'm the Trauma Coordinator for Gwinnett Medical Center. My job is to be the liaison between your family and the physicians and nursing staff who will be participating in Shannon's care during the next few days or weeks."

Immediately, Sue keyed in on her comment:

...the next few days or weeks?... does that mean they now think she will live?...

"Hi, please call me Sue. What can you tell me about her condition?"

"I'm afraid I don't know much more than you do right now. The physicians have spent the day trying to get Shannon stable and make some assessment of her needs in the next day or so. We know she has a severe chest injury that they are watching closely at the moment. Her bladder and spleen repairs look pretty good, but we still haven't been able to determine how bad her head injury is, or if she has any spine damage. The physicians don't want to move her too much until tomorrow. They plan to do some x-rays and a CT scan in the morning. By then we should know a little more."

...it seems like she's been through this before...

"I'm pretty overcome by all the events of the day, and I'm not thinking clearly, so I don't have any specific questions right now."

"The physician in charge of coordinating Shannon's care is Dr. Ken Jenkins, a very competent general surgeon on our staff. He will be sure that the proper specialists are engaged when needed for any specific conditions."

"Tomorrow someone from the business office will be here to see you about insurance coverage and ask you to fill out some forms, and I'll be around to help you in any way that I can. If you have any questions or concerns about Shannon's care, please be sure to call me. I'll get in touch with Dr. Jenkins or the other physicians and get the answers for you. That way, you won't have to call several different places to get information."

"Thank you for your help."

"I know it's been a difficult day for you. We'll do all we can to make the next few days as stress free as we can. I *do* have one important piece of advice for you. *Get as much rest as you can.* You're going to need it when Shannon wakes up! There are plenty of nursing staff here to take care of her tonight. I'd advise you to go home and get some sleep while you can."

...I'll be alright... I'll get through it... it's Shannon I'm worried about...

"Here's my card. I can be reached at that number twenty-four hours a day. Don't hesitate to call me if I can help."

"Thank you, again."

With that, Kathy was gone. She was a tremendous help to us for the next month.

We alternated sitting with Shannon for the next few hours, two at a time. In retrospect, it was a fascinating study in psychology watching how each person spent their time with her. Jennifer was grief stricken. She fought back tears for several hours---for the most part unsuccessfully--- and talked to Shannon just like they were sitting on the floor in the bedroom when they were in junior high school.

Samy was full of 'one-liners', first delivering his lines to Shannon, and then laughing for both of them. He also kept telling her that she was too stubborn to die.

Kelley tried to soothe her, stroking her hand and arm, and telling her to be strong. Neither Brian nor Sue said very much. They were largely lost in thought.

I continued to watch monitors, and paid particularly

31

close attention to the chest drains:

  ...her intracranial pressure is still in the normal range, that's good... blood pressure is down a little, a positive sign... pulse rate has dropped some, *finally*... but still too high... her laparotomy wound seems okay... her collar bone looks terrible... I wonder what they'll do with it? ... I don't know how bad the hip fracture is... her face looks awful... she's going to need extensive surgery... I don't see much change in drainage from the left lung, but it looks like the right one is not draining as much blood... is that a good sign or a bad one? ... her breathing is so labored, *I just don't know*... but we must have hope! ...

  It was dark and quiet in the Intensive Care Unit when we left for Mary Catherine's house, and our home for the next month. It was almost 11:00 p.m., and Shannon's nurse assured us that they would call if there was any change in her condition. Sue and I had terrible feelings of guilt as we left. Here we were, going to sleep safely together in familiar surroundings, while Shannon was in critical condition, lying alone in a strange bed. We didn't know if we'd ever see her alive again.

  I now had a sense of resignation. My bravado of earlier in the day was gone, and I had succumbed to my worst fears. As I rode home, I remembered the warning of many athletic coaches I had as a youth. "Fatigue makes cowards of us all---don't let it get the best of you!"

  As we lay down for a fitful and fearful night of sleep, Sue put her arms around me and cried. She, too, was emotionally spent. "It's going to be okay, she's going to survive," I promised her with as much courage as I could muster."

  "I believe you. *It's just so hard for her*," she replied tearfully. At that moment, neither one of us *really* thought Shannon would survive. We closed our eyes and drifted off to sleep knowing the telephone could ring at any time with the bad news.

Dreams are a strange phenomenon. Sometimes they are good and comforting, and sometimes they are frightening and anxiety producing. And almost always baffling.

There are endless theories about why we dream, what our dreams mean, what their purpose is, how they can be used for therapy, or how they may be harbingers of things to come. We all have them. On this night, one might have reasonably expected a nightmare. But that's not what happened to me. Yes, I awoke several times in a state of anxiety, but the most vivid image of that first night was a flashback to a very happy time in our lives.

Shannon loved gymnastics, and vowed that one day she would 'go to the Olympics'. Yeah, right! Her first hurdle, however, was to figure out how to do a forward roll, a clean cartwheel, a round-off back hand spring on a padded floor---and how to *simply* walk on the four-inch wide balance beam without falling off. Then, to do those things better than all the other aspiring young Nadia Comaneci wannabes.

It was a sunny and cool Saturday morning at the gym at Mountain Brook Elementary School in a southeast suburb of Birmingham, Alabama. There was an excited energy only found when you bring forty-something cute little eight to ten year-old girls together for a competition. They bounded all over the gym in their shiny new team leotards, with multicolor ribbons in their pigtails, ponytails and Dorothy Hamil wedges. It was our first real 'meet', and I, for one, didn't have a clue.

Shannon's coach was Connie Davis. She had the perfect attributes to harness the energy of these budding young stars. She was in her late twenties, was pretty and athletic---having been a gymnast at the University of Alabama, had a pleasant and nurturing personality, and the patience of Job. She organized her troops, reminded them how to march correctly between events, how to 'present' to the judges, and what to do before getting on the vault, bars, beam and floor.

Although parents are not supposed to engage in either discussion or coaching during a competition, it was inevitable that the young charges would look to their parents for comfort and advice. Connie was very tolerant as her legions violated the rule time after time.

Any parent who has followed their child in sport knows that there's a great deal of down time. In gymnastics, you will spend half a day at a meet where your child will actually compete for less than five minutes. And at the lower level competitions, the routines and floor music are the same for all competitors. By the end of the meet, even the casual observer will have memorized the routines on each apparatus and can hum the music without missing a note. It's a grueling process, but one of the memorable times in raising a child.

I don't really remember much about the competition except that Shannon was in the middle of the pack on the beam and bars, and was in the top five or six on the vault. Before she began her turn on the floor exercise, she scampered over to me with a combination of anxiety and anticipation on her face.

"Daddy, I want to win the floor. I need to win. I *have* to win! What should I do?"

"Ask Connie. She's told you exactly what you should do and how to do it."

"No. *I want you to tell me.* You *always* know what to do!"

At that point, I really knew very little about the sport, but I had a feeling I knew what the judges would like. "Honey, all you have to do is smile and jump high!"

Shannon won the floor exercise that day, and my place in her life was secure forever. As I awakened, I

34

realized that the telephone had not rung during the night...
and I felt ready. Today, Sue and I would try to *smile and
jump high.*

---FOUR---

The Big Sleep

Monday, November 13, 1995, 6:10 a.m.

It was approaching dawn as we reached the Intensive Care Unit at Gwinnett Medical Center, and the nursing staff was taking care of last minute housekeeping and paperwork as they prepared for the shift change at 7:00 a.m. Sue and I moved quietly into Shannon's room, looked at monitors, checked the tubes and wires, and closely examined both her severely swollen face and the surgical dressings on her abdomen. Things actually looked encouraging.

During the night the medical staff had reduced both the amount of oxygen she was being given and the pressure with which the ventilator was forcing the life-saving air into her damaged lungs. They had also slowed her respirations to a more normal 20 breaths per minute. Her blood pressure remained relatively high, but it was at least stable. The most immediate concern was still the heavy drainage of blood and mucus from her lungs. On the other hand, her lungs were still able to absorb oxygen, something that Dr. Carter had not expected. Had his initial assessment been correct, Shannon would likely have expired by now.

"Good morning, Mr. and Mrs. Lloyd. Shannon had a restful night. I hope you did too." We turned to see her night nurse as she entered the room. "She's still critical, but I think there's reason for hope. Dr. Jenkins will be here in the next couple of hours, and he can tell you what the plan is for today." Her tone and optimism were as heartening as the sun that now began peeking through the windows.

Around 8:30 a.m., a tall, pleasant appearing physician ambled into the ICU. A quick look at the name on his white coat told us that it was indeed, Ken Jenkins, M.D. We also knew immediately that we were going to like him.

"I'm Ken Jenkins, and I'll be directing Shannon's care for as long as she's here."

Good morning, I'm Don Lloyd. We appreciate your help."

"Hi, Dr. Jenkins, I'm Sue. Thanks for all you did yesterday for Shannon."

In the next few minutes, Dr. Jenkins carefully told us everything he knew about Shannon's condition. He apologized for not being able to give us more definitive answers to our questions, but painstakingly reviewed the plans for the day and the foreseeable future. First, she needed some neck, spine and pelvic x-rays to see if she had any fractures that had not yet been detected. She was also going to need a CT scan of her head to assess the extent of her facial injuries and determine the severity of her head trauma. He told us that Dr. Curtis Roe, a neurosurgeon, would be by to see us once the results of the CT scan were available. It was our first slight indication that we were going to have to contend with a brain injury.

Dr. Jenkins was a general surgeon in his mid-forties who had trained at Emory University. As he patiently talked with us, I thought how fortunate we were to have such a competent and caring physician advocate:

...Emory has a reputation for excellence, and Dr. Jenkins certainly confirms that... his demeanor is calm and sincere... I know he's busy, but he doesn't seem rushed... and he's talking *with* us, not down to us... I *like* him...

As the morning wore on, Kelley and Brian arrived, along with Shannon's grandparents and many of their church congregation. Also, more of Shannon's friends from across the Southeast. The telephone was now ringing almost constantly. Frankly, the sheer number of well-wishers astounded us.

The first major event of the day came around 11:00 a.m. when the nursing staff began preparing Shannon for transport to the Radiology Department for her x-rays and CT scan. She had not been moved significantly on Sunday because the medical staff feared that she would again become unstable.

The nurses were very cautious as they disconnected some of the monitors and piled the other ones on the bed as they wheeled Shannon out of the Unit for her destination a couple of floors away. She tolerated the jostling and movement without incident.

As the doors to the ICU opened and Shannon's bed emerged, the throngs of people present naturally wanted to see what she looked like. I can't adequately describe the depth of shock and horror displayed as she passed by the waiting area. It was cemetery quiet as many of those present just stared in disbelief. Some of her friends simply turned away and cried, some hugged one another, and a few others followed her intently with their eyes. While they had all known intellectually that the situation was critical, this parade of sorts captured them emotionally. It was real... *Shannon might actually die!*

All of a sudden the room began to roar as people began comparing notes. They talked about her face, the tubes, probes and monitors... and the fact that she was totally unresponsive. This led to the inevitable story telling and reminiscing that happens when one looks back on their life with old friends.

"Do ya'll remember Homecoming our senior year at Valley?" asked Jennifer rhetorically. "We used my garage to decorate the float... Shannon fell and got paint all over herself... then got mad because we laughed at her? Then she got even by throwing paint all over us? That was a blast."

"That sounds like her, alright," added Samy with a hearty laugh. "She always likes to be the one to start something, claiming that it's one of her *charming* personality traits! She didn't change much from high school to college, did she?" The stories continued for several hours as they kept vigil. Talking about the *good times* helped lighten the mood and lessen the emotional pain.

Shannon was returned to the Intensive Care Unit about 12:30 p.m. with her condition unchanged. We once again assessed the situation and concluded that she had held her own during the procedures. This led to the second major event of the day. We learned that Shannon was to be moved to a larger ICU room and placed in a 'rescue bed'. This was the first definitive indication to us that the doctors believed she might have a chance to survive.

A 'rescue bed' is essentially a motorized hospital bed that constantly rocks from side to side. The purpose of the perpetual movement is to facilitate the circulation of fluids in the body of a patient who cannot move on their own. It's used in the treatment of the spinal cord injured, head trauma patients, stroke victims, or any other patients who are immobile.

Since this was the first time the hospital had used a 'rescue bed', it had to be ordered from a medical supply company and arrived by truck from the supplier around noon. Sue and I actually helped the nursing staff unpack and prepare the 'rescue bed' for use. It was also the first time we had laughed since the fateful telephone call as we collectively tried to figure out how fast the contraption should sway and how much tilt was appropriate.

I was the guinea pig, as I hopped in the bed and they turned on the juice. The first settings were so fast, and had so much tilt, that I was almost thrown out of the bed. We all had a good laugh as I struggled to stay in the semi-crib. After a few adjustments, we felt that we had arrived at the proper settings.

As Sue and I left the ICU while the staff re-situated Shannon, it occurred to us that *we now actually believed* she was going to survive. We were still conscious of the ARDS risk, but it seemed to us that if her lungs were going to harden, they would have begun to do so by now. The evidence suggested to us that she was going to overcome that hurdle. There was still no official indication from the nursing staff or physicians that our assessment was correct. Still, we felt some sense of confidence.

The third significant event of the day came a few minutes after 3:00 p.m. when Dr. Curtis Roe, the neurosurgeon assigned to the case, arrived with the results of the x-rays and CT scans. While there were multiple facial fractures, there was no damage to her neck or back. This allowed them to remove the cervical collar. They confirmed the suspected hairline fracture to her left hip, which would not require any immediate treatment. Surprisingly enough, this slight injury was to cause Shannon and the family much grief in the next three or four months.

Dr. Roe told us that her CT scan was clear except for a minor bleed in the right upper posterior portion of Shannon's brain. He believed it would resolve by itself, but that we may see some minor memory disturbance later. We quizzed him about when she might awake from her coma, and he casually replied that it might be a couple of days or a couple of weeks. He simply didn't seem that concerned. We, unfortunately, didn't know enough to be as bothered as we should have been. While we liked his optimism, he seemed preoccupied and rushed.

Shortly after Dr. Roe left, another physician who we didn't know strutted into the ICU Unit. Here was a young man with a *very* comfortable ego. It was Dr. Willard Thompson Leonare, a maxillofacial surgeon. It would be his job to repair the extensive damage to Shannon's face.

"Good afternoon, I'm Tom Leonare (*pronounced len-air*). My job is to make your daughter pretty again!" He then went straight to the bedside and began to carefully examine every inch of her face. As he did so, he explained what he was seeing.

"Your daughter has two shock fractures to her eye orbits... the bones that support and keep the eyes in place. Most likely the orbits just cracked from the centrifugal force of stopping so suddenly. The bones in her nose have literally been destroyed. We won't be able to do anything about that now, but we can take care of that in a later surgery. She has multiple fractures of the bones in her cheeks, with the most damage to the left side where she obviously hit the windshield or frame of the car. Her jaw is also broken in several places. Her mouth and teeth seem to be in good shape... I don't see any that are missing or broken. We'll try to schedule her for surgery on Thursday. Do you have any questions?"

By this time, I was totally absorbed by my thoughts:
...this is bad---*really bad!*... she'll never look the same again... she's going to have pocked marked scars all over the left side of her face where the shards of glass were imbedded... her nose is smashed... her beautiful high cheekbones are gone... a broken jaw, too?... *oh, me*... what are we going to do? ...

While I may have been preoccupied, Sue was not. She was ready for some answers. "Dr. Leonare, can you repair all this damage?"

"I certainly can. It may take awhile, but I'll fix her up as good as new." He had absolutely no doubt.

"Well, how long will it take?"

"Oh, probably eight to ten hours. I won't know that until we get started."

"How bad will the scars be?" *She had just asked him the wrong question.*

42

Dr. Leonare slowly rose from his chair, looked down at Sue with a mock look of disgust, and responded in his most indignant tone. "Mrs. Lloyd, *my patients don't have scars*! I want you to bring me a recent full facial photograph to use as a reference. I'll make her look just like that again." He then turned and left the room.

As Tom Leonare left, he turned and smiled. "I'll see you tomorrow, and we'll finalize the surgery date. And don't forget the photograph."

Sue and I just looked at one another with both a sense of optimism and bewilderment. "I only hope he's as good as he *thinks he is*," I muttered to her in amazement.

As the day was drawing to a close, we felt that some progress had been made. The talk of death and dying subsided as we began contemplating the impending surgeries, treatments and rehabilitation to come. It was also necessary to turn our attention to the logistical issues that surrounded a lengthy hospital stay in a town almost three hundred miles from home.

We had to get clothing, Kelley still had to complete classes at Middle Tennessee State University, and I had both Clinic and Medical Group Management Association duties to attend to. We were also now faced with another stark reality. How were we going to pay for all this?

It was decided that Kelley and I would return to Murfreesboro and try to clear the decks for the next few days until we had a clearer picture of what the longer term looked like. We would take care of important tasks and try to get back as soon as we could. When we were convinced that Shannon was stable, Kelley and I left for home. Sue and Brian stayed until 10:30 p.m. A critical day had passed, and the family had remained intact.

❖❖❖

Tuesday morning started with a telephone call to the hospital. Shannon had rested well, and her vital signs looked much more normal. Particularly encouraging was the marked decrease in lung drainage, especially on the right side.

It became a day of watchful waiting for Sue, her parents, and a few friends. Many of those who had been at the hospital had to get back to their lives, and the waiting room and hospital corridors became much more subdued and clinical. Samy left to return to South Carolina, but vowed to be back as soon as he could make alternative arrangements for his medical school exams. His absence made the hospital seem even more reserved and impersonal.

Meanwhile, Kelley and I conducted our required business, packed some clothes, and left Murfreesboro around 11:00 a.m. We arrived back at the hospital just after 4:00 p.m. Things looked good. We had weathered the initial shock of the accident, had gotten some positive feedback from physicians and staff, and felt that the situation was under control for now. We certainly weren't overconfident, but we increasingly felt that time was on our side.

As the angst of the trauma subsided, we began to have some time to think about the future. While Shannon had survived the initial ordeal, there were still many immediate dangers to confront. She was in a coma. When she would regain consciousness was an open question. For us, it wasn't a matter of *if* she would awaken...but *when.*

Then there were worries related to her impending facial surgery, possible infection at her many wound and needle sites, permanent lung and bladder function, and possible feeding tube complications. We also began to have questions about how to manage the long-term effects that might remain after she regained consciousness. We still had no real concept of what was to come, however.

In the first few hours after the accident, our only goal was to save Shannon's life. We wanted everyone to do whatever was necessary to save her and relieve her pain. Now, with some time to think, our attention turned to economics. We knew the cost of the ordeal would be substantial, and we knew we were going to have to figure out a way to pay for it. Her insurance should take care of most of it, right? Not in this case... you see, Shannon didn't have any health insurance.

Shannon's lack of insurance was another dramatic shock for us. She wasn't eligible for our insurance plan because she was no longer a student, and we had been told that she was enrolled in her company's plan. Through a clerical error, her employer had misplaced her application for insurance, and Shannon had failed to follow up to be sure her coverage was in effect. Another of life's ironies. I had spent a working lifetime in medicine, and yet my own daughter had no health insurance. It *literally* added insult to injury.

Technically, Sue and I had no economic responsibility because Shannon was an adult, living on her own. However, we felt an obligation to see that everyone who participated in Shannon's care was paid. It was an overpowering thought at the time, and a struggle for several years afterward.

Wednesday was a day of alternating anticipation and frustration. After consultation with Dr. Jenkins and Dr. Roe, Dr. Leonare had decided to do Shannon's facial surgery sooner rather than later. Their thinking was that they did not want to have to anesthetize her for eight to ten hours just as she was waking up from a coma. Now time was of the essence.

The nursing staff reported that Shannon had moved her hands and feet slightly during the night... and actually blinked her eyes once or twice in the early morning. After a rather ponderous day on Tuesday, events were again moving at warp speed.

Just as they were getting ready to take her to surgery, there was a flurry of activity. Shannon acted as though she was trying to get up, and actually opened her eyes and looked straight at me for a brief instant. One can only imagine the emotions I felt. Then, before I knew it, she was headed down the hall toward the operating room.

The next several hours were torturous. We took some telephone calls, talked quietly with family members, and just sat anxiously awaiting word from the operating room. Our first report came from a nurse around 5:00 p.m.

"Mrs. Lloyd, Dr. Leonare started the surgery at 1:30 p.m. He is making good progress. Shannon is tolerating the procedure well. I'll see you again in a couple of hours. Don't worry... Dr. Leonare is the *best*." She then disappeared as abruptly as she arrived.

More friends and family started arriving after the dinner hour, and the corridors again came alive. More Shannon 'war stories', more laughter, and much tension. The telephone rang at 7:40 p.m. It was the nurse from the operating room.

"Shannon's doing fine. Dr. Leonare thinks it will be another hour or so before he finishes. He'll come out to see you when he's through. Again, try not to worry... she's in no pain, and the repairs are going well."

We were pleased with the report, but after six and a half hours under anesthesia, we were now openly wondering about the after-effects of being sedated for such a long period. How much more could she take?

It was 9:20 p.m. when Dr. Tom Leonare emerged from the operating suite door. He was soaked with sweat and beaming from ear to ear. As they say, a picture is worth a thousand words. And the picture was good.

"The surgery went very well. Some of her injuries

weren't as bad as I first thought. Shannon's nose and eye orbits fell nicely back into place. She shouldn't have any trouble with her sight. Her left cheekbones were pretty well demolished, but we used titanium plates to reform them, as well as the left mandible. We also plated her left temple and..."

I don't remember how long he talked because I slipped into deep thought as he described the procedure in detail:

...shaved her head... cut her from ear to ear... peeled her face down to access the bones?... *gruesome...* **rebuilt her cheekbones... and her jaw... arch bars on her teeth... couldn't do anything with her nose because of the feeding tube... will need further surgery to repair the nose... what a mess! ...**

"...it will take some time, but she'll be as pretty as ever. Do you have any questions?"

We were so dumbfounded by his detailed description that all we could manage was a weak 'thank you'.

"Well then. I'll see you tomorrow." His gait told the story as he walked down the hall. He was a very self-satisfied man!

As we basked in the success of the facial surgery, and waited for Shannon to be returned to the ICU, another critical issue arose, and we were suddenly back on the down side of the roller coaster. Dr. Jenkins had consulted a gastroenterologist, Dr. Carl McCutcheon, to discuss nutrition and long term feeding. Apparently, they felt that Shannon would not be able to feed herself for some time to come---*if ever*!

This assessment was devastating, and we were unwilling to accept it as fact until we had more information and a fair chance to evaluate the options. Just moments before, we were feeling that things were finally moving in a positive direction... and now this!

One of the initial actions taken in the emergency room on Sunday morning was the insertion of a nasogastric, or NG Tube, for short term feeding. Now that it looked like Shannon might survive, Dr. McCutcheon wanted to replace the NG Tube with a more permanent feeding mechanism called a jejeunostomy, or J-tube.

This tube was to be inserted directly through the abdomen into Shannon's small intestine. It would allow the feedings to by-pass her mouth and upper intestines. It was explained to us that once placed, the J-Tube would have to remain for at least six to eight weeks, and Shannon would be unable to attempt to take food by mouth during this period. We thought this was too drastic a measure.

After some discussion with both Dr. Jenkins and Dr. McCutcheon, we decided on a less drastic type feeding tube that would allow Shannon to take nourishment either from a tube placed directly into the stomach or by mouth. Sue and I felt that this gave us some flexibility to try oral feedings relatively soon after Shannon woke up rather than having to wait several weeks or months. It was finally agreed that Dr. Jenkins and Dr. McCutcheon would place a gastrostomy, or G-Tube, directly into Shannon's stomach on Thursday.

The G-Tube, also commonly called a PEG, would allow a nutritional formula to be funneled into Shannon's stomach continuously by a feeding pump or manually by the nurse several times a day, as appropriate. She would also be able to take food by mouth. If and when she was able to gain enough sustenance by eating normally, the PEG could be removed. We didn't know whether or not it was the right decision, but it was our best judgment, given what we knew then. We knew that only time would tell.

❖❖❖

Thursday was day five of the ordeal, and we had now found our routine. We would arrive early at the hospital and evaluate how the night went; look at monitors, IVs, drains and tubes; talk with nursing staff and any physicians we could find; prepare for the day's tests, treatments or assessments; and brace ourselves for the unexpected, but inevitable, event of the day.

The night had gone well. So well, in fact, that the settings on the ventilator had again been reduced significantly. Shannon was breathing substantially on her own, and was showing signs of restlessness. The tone for the day was set shortly after we arrived at the hospital.

The ICU waiting room was small... perhaps measuring twelve by fourteen feet. There were seats for no more than fifteen people. As a result, families and friends of patients in the ICU would also set up camp in the corridor. When there were several patients in the Unit, the hallway got very congested and loud.

On this morning, however, it was quiet and I was sitting in a strategic position behind an old wooden desk in a corner of the corridor. It was just outside the entrance to the surgery suite on one side, the ICU door on the other side, and the waiting room on the third side. It was a good place to write the journal I was keeping, and an excellent position from which I could survey all the activity or spot physicians entering the floor.

As I was writing, I heard a noise at the far end of the corridor, approximately a hundred feet away. I looked up to see Dr. Carter, the pulmonologist who had first greeted us on Sunday morning. He caught a glimpse of me at the same time. What happened next not only surprised me, but also changed my mind about 'Dr. All Business'. He began hippity-hopping down the hallway waving x-rays in the air.

"Her lungs are clearing... her lungs are clearing... her lungs are clearing!" he yelled.

49

By the time he got to me, he was so out of breath I thought I was going to have to resuscitate him!

"Mr. Lloyd, I never thought I'd see this. Your daughter's lungs are improving at a remarkable rate. I've never seen anything like it! It looks like she's going to regain full lung function in a few days, and we'll be able to take her off the ventilator. It's a miracle!"

I was just as ecstatic as he was... but I wasn't surprised. "Thanks for the great news. I knew if there was any chance at all, she would be the one to do it. She was a *very determined* athlete!"

Dr. Carter just smiled, said goodbye and went into the Unit. I sat pensively for a moment, thinking about my first encounter with him. Upon reflection, I realized that his initial assessment on Sunday morning was intended to regulate our expectations. In the medical profession, it's known as 'crepe hanging'.

There is nothing worse than giving a family false hope, only to have to report the patient's demise later. It's always better to paint a gloomy picture and be pleasantly surprised if the patient beats the odds. When outcomes exceed expectations, there is plenty of cause to celebrate. Dr. Carter indeed cared, and it was his day of triumph.

I felt good, and was absolutely convinced that the worst was over. It seemed just a matter of time before Shannon would be off the ventilator and would wake up from her coma.

Around noon, they wheeled Shannon to the operating room to insert the PEG. It took less than an hour. Shannon's housemates, Cassie Clark and Martha Burks, arrived just as Shannon was being brought back to the Unit. Once we were convinced that all was well, Sue, Brian, Kelley and I actually left the hospital to get lunch while Cassie and Martha stood watch.

The waiting room and corridor began filling up with friends and family by mid-afternoon. Samy had also returned, and the hospital came alive again. Throughout the day, we took turns sitting with Shannon, and began what turned out to be hours of 'fiddling' with everything in sight. This was all done in preparation for her waking up in the next day or two.

We knew Shannon would be frightened when she became aware of her surroundings and saw all the tubes, wires and probes. Accordingly, we tried to do everything we could to anticipate anything that might upset or irritate her. Sue and Kelley cleaned her eyes, scalp, hands, feet, IV sites, and anything else they could get to. We organized the tubes that had heretofore been haphazardly draped on various parts of the bed. And we put pictures of Shannon and her friends on the nightstand.

We chuckled as we prepared for Shannon's return, because it reminded us of how we used to treat her before gymnastics meets. The older Shannon got... and the more successful she became, the more she began turning into a supreme primadonna. In the few days leading up to a competition, we literally did everything we could to please her so she wouldn't get distracted or upset.

It seemed that even the most inconsequential misstep would agitate her, so we gave her foods she liked, let her watch her favorite television programs, and generally just kept out of her way. As one can imagine, this got old after awhile. However, this experience helped us understand her psyche so well that it provided a useful foundation for coaching her through her brain injury recovery.

Dr. Leonare came by to check on Shannon after dinner, and when he discovered that Samy was a medical student he immediately went into a 'teaching mode' and began explaining in great detail everything he did to Shannon's face. It was quite an education for all of us.

Samy was mesmerized. It was right up his alley.

As the day drew to a close, we were sure that Shannon was now on the verge of waking up. We talked about when she would start responding to verbal commands, when she would open her eyes, and what she would say to us. It turned into a contest.

"I think her first real response will be at 8:30 pm on Friday," avowed Samy.

"You're way off, Samy," chided Kelley. "I'll bet it's more like Saturday at noon."

"Your both wrong," I observed. "I'm pretty sure it will be late on Sunday. Probably around dinner time."

"I'll bet that Samy's closer to being right. I think she'll show signs of coming back to us by 6:30 tomorrow night."

As it turned out, Sue was correct... it was late on Friday afternoon that Shannon began to squeeze a hand on command. We went home on Thursday night anxious for Friday to come.

The next three days were full of alternating periods of anticipation, disappointment and impatience. By Friday, Shannon was becoming very active. She seemed concerned with the little things like the rocking of the trauma bed, the restraints on her arms, the various tubes and wires penetrating her body, and the ventilator. While she was still unconscious, it was clear that she wanted to get out of the bed.

By midday on Friday, Shannon was largely breathing on her own. The ventilator was still in place to add pressure to her lungs to keep them expanded longer so she could absorb more oxygen. The doctors planned to remove the life support machine on Saturday or Sunday. The swelling in her face from the surgery was subsiding nicely, and she began to look less like a lopsided basketball and more like a human being. It was simply a matter of time before her swollen eyes would improve enough for her to open them.

Shannon had spiked a slight fever on Thursday, which is not particularly unusual after a trauma or surgery, but by Friday it was over 101 degrees. We learned from blood cultures that she had an infection. It was a worrisome setback. The etiology of the bacteria was the site of the central line in her chest on the upper left side. The line was replaced and she was put on antibiotics.

The fallout from the episode was a decision to begin a month-long parade of changing IVs every three or four days to avoid both infection and inflammation at the various needle sites. Each exchange caused pain, and we wondered how much more Shannon could endure.

The weekend brought a whole host of new and return visitors from all over the Southeast. It turned into a real episode of 'This is Your Life', with so many childhood, college and graduate school friends in one place at the same time. In fact, there were so many people crowded into the waiting room and corridor that it became pure bedlam. It got so loud that hospital officials had to ask the visitors to disburse several times.

The show of love and support was both remarkable and humbling. As I sat at my wooden desk watching the action, I was overwhelmed with emotion. My mind wandered and I wished I could trade places with Shannon so she could enjoy the company of her lifetime of friends.

My thoughts at the time were recorded in my journal:

...Shannon, I wanted to be sure to let you know how important you are to me. Any of us would have traded places with you to spare you the pain and frustration that you're feeling, but you and I have always had that special 'soul bond', *and I really feel for you.* **I wanted to be in that bed instead of you because you have so much life yet to live. You are very precious to us as a family; and to many friends in**

many places... we can't help but believe that you'll be fine in time, but you'll have to be tough and strong. I *know* you can do it! I'm counting on it...

During the weekend, there were several reports that Shannon had blinked her eyes. Unfortunately, I was never there to verify it. Because she was becoming so active and was improving at a comfortable pace, Shannon was removed from the trauma bed and placed in a regular hospital bed on Sunday. Early in the day her chest drains had been removed and the ventilator had been turned off, although the tube remained in place as a precaution.

As Sunday evening drew to a close, I returned to Tennessee to catch up on events at work, confident that the worst was finally over. We expected setbacks, but I was sure we could cope with whatever the future would bring. I could not have been more wrong.

To me, the most significant and indelible memory of the first week was not a medical treatment, surgery or therapy... but rather the imprint Shannon left on those who saw the severity of her injuries.

Initially, only the immediate family, Samy and Jennifer were allowed into the ICU to see her. Others caught a glimpse of Shannon as she was being taken to the surgery suite. Later when she was more stable, I took more friends and family back into the ICU so they could see the full picture for themselves. That's when the *real* impact of the event struck home.

The older family members were deeply distressed, both for Shannon and us... *as well as for themselves and their own children.* It was very sobering to see this once vibrant young woman lying near death. Her young adult friends and cousins felt the ultimate devastation, however. Without exception, each one of them was shocked and mortified by the sight of Shannon lying unconscious in a rotating bed, with the seemingly endless number of tubes and wires penetrating her body. The tears flowed freely as they all saw themselves in that bed... *and it wasn't a comforting thought.*

My most lasting impression of their reactions came from my brother's twenty-three year old son, Brent. A happy-go-lucky college student at Vanderbilt, he stood over Shannon's bed at his full height of six feet three inches. He said nothing as I lectured him about the consequences of bad choices, but I knew he understood. He simply closed his eyes as the tears streamed down his face. He was crushed... just like the rest of us!

---FIVE---

The Awakening

Monday, November 20, 1995, 7:14 a.m. *Ring...ring...ring...*

"Hello, this is Dr. LaRoche. Yes he is...just a moment. Don, it's for you... it's your wife."

So it was... in the middle of a meeting of the Board of Directors of the Murfreesboro Medical Clinic, when the most important news of my life came to me. Shannon was now somewhat conscious, and she at least recognized Sue and Kelley. The awakening we had all prayed for was now beginning. It was also my fiftieth birthday.

The eyes of all seven physicians and three administrative colleagues were on me as I reached for the telephone.

"Hello... is everything alright?"

"Yes. Everything's fine. Shannon is waking up. She seems to know us, but she's pretty confused about where she is."

"Does she still have the breathing tube in?"

"Yes. While she's breathing on her own, they're still reluctant to take it out until her blood gasses look a little better. The nurse says she's ready, but the doctors want to wait a little longer."

"So she can't speak."

"Not clearly, but she did say Mom and Kelley when we asked her who we were. It was garbled, but she *did* recognize us. When are you coming back?"

"I had planned to return tomorrow, but I'll see if I can finish some things here and leave in the late afternoon. I should be there by 8:00 or 9:00 p.m. Thanks for the news, honey."

Thus the next phase of our long journey had begun. Throughout the day, the nursing staff kept close watch on Shannon. Sue and Kelley talked to her constantly, not wanting her to close her eyes or drift back into sleep. In spite of their efforts, Shannon floated in and out of consciousness throughout the day.

During the times that Shannon was awake, Sue, Kelley, and the nursing staff would talk to her and try to get her to obey simple commands. Sometimes she was able to comply, and at other times she just stared blankly at the ceiling. One thing was clear... Shannon did not like all the tubes and wires, particularly the one down her throat. After she reached for it once, Sue realized that she and Kelley would have to hold her hands constantly to keep her from pulling one or more of the tubes out.

Sometime in the late morning, Kathy Dunbar, the Trauma Coordinator, came in to see how Shannon was doing. She was appalled that the breathing tube was still in place, and vowed to 'pitch a fit' until it was removed. First, however, she needed to test Shannon's ability to respond. She passed, and Kathy was off like a shot to fulfill her promise.

Now that Shannon was semi-conscious, she was very reactive to pain. Every time she was moved, her brow would furrow, her eyes would sharpen, and she would cry out. It was hard to watch. It was, however, necessary to begin moving her so that physical therapy could begin as soon as possible.

During my many years in health care, I have seen any number of critically ill or injured patients. The obvious conclusion one draws when looking at recovery rates is that young people heal faster and more completely than older ones. That's certainly to be expected. A second, and not so apparent, observation is that no matter what the age, an active patient recovers much more quickly than a sedentary one. In fact, the body deteriorates at an astonishingly rapid rate if the patient remains prone.

I had first hand experience with this phenomenon after my seventy-one year old mother fell and broke her hip a few years before. In a ten-day period from the time of her fall until her surgery and subsequent death, she quickly became so feeble that her body frame simply couldn't support her. The lesson for caregivers is that patients must get up as soon as possible... whether it's painful or not.

Before the day was through, Shannon had a visit from two physical therapists, Cindi and Laura. They methodically moved and massaged her extremities, shifted her in the bed, and sat her up so they could assess her strength and coordination. Shannon protested. In spite of her unsteadiness, they pressed on. We learned that this was only the beginning of what would turn out to be often chaotic and tumultuous therapy sessions.

The two young therapists established from their initial visit that they were probably in store for some verbal and physical abuse throughout the course of treatment. They remained unfazed, however, and told us that this kind of behavior was typical of brain injury cases.

Once Shannon was alert enough to follow simple commands with regularity, Sue tried to explain to her that she had been in an automobile accident, had some bad injuries, and had been asleep for nine days. It was clear from her reactions, however, that she was bewildered and probably couldn't comprehend what she was being told. Sue and Kelley continually reassured her that she would be fine in time. She responded each time by moving her head side to side as if to say, "No, I won't."

At approximately 5:00 p.m., one of the nurses came in to remove the breathing tube. Shannon wanted it removed, but was terrified that she wouldn't be able to breathe without it. Mother and sister again assured her that all would be fine... even though they were just as apprehensive as she was. The ventilator tube was pulled and replaced with an oxygen mask. Shannon didn't like that any better, but she could now at least talk... or attempt to talk.

I suspect that most people have the same concept of coma recovery that I did prior to our direct experience with it. The patient is unconscious for days, weeks or even months, then suddenly awakens with a clear head and asks, "Where am I? How long was I out? Boy, it's good to see you!" Well, that's not exactly what happens. The patient awakens very slowly, and *if* he or she can actually speak, the words will likely be unintelligible or incoherent at best. Much of that depends on what part of the brain has been injured.

According to the National Institutes of Health, there are more than 700,000 brain injuries each year in the United States. They occur when the victim's head is impacted by a blunt or piercing force such as an automobile dashboard or windshield, a fall to the ground off a ladder, a violent assault, or even a bullet wound.

The injury may be minimal, as in a mild concussion, or it may be completely debilitating, as in the case of President Reagan's Press Secretary, James Brady. The extent and duration of the injury depends on a variety of factors, such as what kind of force caused the injury, where the force occurred, how powerful the force was, how old or healthy the individual is, or any number of other influences. The problem that doctors and families face is that it's so hard to tell how bad the injury is because the damage isn't readily visible.

Yes, there are scans of all sorts to help pinpoint the damaged areas, but because each brain is different, it's difficult to assess the real scope of the injury in any one individual. In spite of their heroic efforts, physicians simply can't forecast the course of recovery in severely injured patients any better than pundits can predict the outcome of sporting events or elections.

More than 200,000 people die from head injuries annually, and another 500,000 or so require hospitalization. Of the brain injury survivors, approximately ten percent or 50,000 victims have mild to moderate long-term effects. Another forty percent or 200,000 have permanent debilitating effects that require close supervision or institutionalization for life. We, of course, did not know this as Shannon was coming back to life.

As the evening progressed, Shannon became more aware of her surroundings. Sue and Kelley talked to her about her friends and generally tried to reassure her that she would eventually be okay. Her responses were muted, but nonetheless, positive. Just when things looked like they were going well, Shannon started to exhibit signs of confusion and panic. Suddenly her ability to speak and control motor movements deteriorated badly.

For the first few moments after the ventilator tube was removed, Shannon seemed to be able to speak somewhat intelligibly, but now she was regressing to the point that communication became almost impossible. She could now barely speak; her words were slurred, and the words she did speak seemed inappropriate and incoherent.

While the nurse didn't seem overly concerned about the changing conditions, Sue and Kelley certainly did. The promising beginning had turned sour. What happened? Nothing unusual, according to the experts. While this may have been disconcerting, it was apparently part of the normal awakening process. After a few minutes of struggle, Shannon abruptly lapsed into a deep sleep.

The pattern quickly revealed itself when Shannon woke up after a couple of hours of sleep. She was once more at least somewhat coherent, and much more cooperative. *Another important lesson.* Sleep does indeed refresh the brain. We experienced this phenomenon, although less dramatically, again and again for many months. Clearly, brain rest is very important to head injury victims, and it became apparent over time that when she was tired, Shannon just couldn't communicate effectively.

Human behavior is baffling under the most normal of circumstances, but predicting it in the brain injured is almost impossible. In Shannon's case, it was volatile and erratic. She was alternately pleasant and agreeable, angry and abusive, determined and aggressive, cooperative and compliant, frightened and withdrawn, then just silent. In the next month we experienced all of these conflicting emotions… and more.

The exhausting day drew to a close just after 9:00 p.m. when I arrived back at the hospital. I was excited but apprehensive as I walked back into the ICU room. Sue and Kelley were smiling, Shannon's eyes were wide open and I was bursting with emotion.

"Shannon, do you know who that is?" Sue asked.

"Brian," she answered weakly.

My heart was broken. At that moment, I realized the road ahead was going to be long and demanding… *and who knew where it would end.*

Tuesday, November 21 was a big day. It was time to leave the Intensive Care Unit behind, and move to a private room on the surgery floor. Unbeknownst to us, Room 616 would become a torture chamber for everybody involved in Shannon's care.

The first day began innocently enough. We had meetings with the nursing staff, as well as occupational, physical and speech therapists to discuss immediate and long-term care protocols. They gave us instructions about how to tend to her hygiene needs, the importance of mental stimulation... tempered by appropriate rest periods, the need to get her out of bed soon, and the kind of behaviors we might expect from a head injury victim.

While we were obviously pleased that Shannon's level of awareness had improved, it brought with it a whole new set of problems. She had to be supervised constantly to keep her from pulling at her tubes or trying to get up before she was strong enough to support herself again. She was now a handful.

During the day she was confused, restless and agitated.   At times she seemed to understand her surroundings, but most of the time she was just plain baffled by everything. She seemed to know her family, but we sensed that she comprehended little else.   That impression was confirmed by mid-afternoon.

Like most young girls, Shannon had always been very meticulous about her appearance. She would spend an inordinate amount of time choosing her clothes each day, fixing her hair and make-up, and would be appalled at the slightest imperfection. When we arrived in the sixth floor room, what did we see but a giant mirror on the wall a few feet away from her bed.

We were sure that when she saw herself in the mirror she would be completely destroyed. It didn't take long before she looked squarely into the mirror... and had absolutely no reaction. The truth is, she probably didn't even know the reflection in the mirror was her! If she did, she just didn't care.

During the day, several caregivers visited Shannon. Some were optimistic about her long-term prognosis, and others were less confident.   Two of the late afternoon visitors were representatives from Jerome Grant Rehabilitation Hospital, a facility located about twenty-miles away from the Gwinnett Medical Center.   They suggested that Shannon would need to be transferred to their facility in a couple of weeks for long-term therapy. They indicated that someone would be back the next couple of days to help us make arrangements for the transfer. Sue was crushed. Once again, I was a disbeliever. *I didn't believe for a minute that Shannon was going to need extended custodial care.*

A visit from the Neurosurgeon, Dr. Roe, made us feel better. He was as confident of her recovery as Dr. Leonare was of his facial surgery. We just prayed that he was right. We were still somewhat shaken as Dr. Roe left, but we felt that a good night's sleep and the beginning of intensive therapy the next day would be just the right avenue to recovery.

Kelley and I volunteered to stay the first night with Shannon. As she fell asleep just after dark, we looked at her and cried. It had been ten days since the accident, and here was my daughter and Kelley's sister, still unable to speak coherently, unable to control any fine motor movements, and unaware of her surroundings.

She still had two IVs in each arm, a Foley catheter in her bladder, a rectal tube, an abdominal drain, a feeding tube in her stomach, an oxygen mask over her nose and mouth, and was hooked up to an electrocardiograph (ECG monitor). Her head was shaved from mid scalp forward; she had over thirty large metal staples in her head from ear to ear holding together the surgical wound; and she had clearly lost ten to fifteen pounds. It was a pathetic sight.

Kelley and I only had a short time to feel sorry for her, however, because the respite was about to end. After perhaps an hour, Shannon awakened and was very disoriented. She was unable to comprehend where she was or who we were. She wanted to get up. She tried to pull out the feeding tube. She tried to unhook the ECG wires. She cried out for help. She cried out in pain. Shannon was in the middle of her worst nightmare...and she was determined to take us with her.

In short... it was the night from *Hell*. After a couple of hours of struggle, Kelley and I devised a plan of action. We positioned ourselves on either side of the bed, and each grabbed one of Shannon's hands. Neither of us was to let go of that hand for more than an instant for the next ten hours. We sat in an auditorium chair, laid our heads on the side of the bed... and kept a firm grip on Shannon's hand or arm. When she began to squirm, we'd tighten our grip. When she tried to get up, we'd spring to our feet and wrestle her back down. Shannon would yell, and we would try to calm her down. All to no avail.

Occasionally we would gain control and Shannon would fall into a deep sleep, only to have a nurse come in the room, turn on the light and poke, probe or stick her with a needle. The process would then begin all over again. By the time Sue arrived at 8:30 a.m., Kelley and I were demoralized and exhausted.

When we described the night to Sue, she gave us a look that was all too familiar. She thought we were exaggerating. She later found out differently. Kelley and I left to go clean up and get some rest. Sue and her sister, Kim, then took over for much of the day.

The ebb and flow of emotions that we had felt in the first ten days, and would feel periodically for several years, was never more evident than on this Wednesday. Sue was developing an eye infection, and was constantly wiping the drainage from her eyes. It looked like she was crying much of the time. In reality, she was fearful that if the nurses discovered her ailment, she would be asked to leave, so she was content to let them think she was just a fretting mother constantly wiping tears from her eyes. Unfortunately, the tears became authentic by late morning.

"Good morning, Mrs. Lloyd. I'm Melissa Anderson, and I'm a Clinical Evaluator from the Rehab Division of the North Georgia Health System. I wanted to spend a few minutes with you to review the services we offer at our Jerome Grant Facility, and talk about Shannon's transfer in the next couple of weeks."

Sue was flabbergasted, and wasn't mentally prepared to discuss the subject of long-term rehabilitation yet. Ms. Anderson asked her to come down the hall to a small office where they could talk privately. Kim accompanied her while a floor nurse stayed with Shannon.

"I know this is difficult for you," continued Ms. Anderson. "And I want to assure you that we'll do everything we can to give Shannon every chance possible to regain *some* ability to take care of herself in the future." Sue and Kim just looked at each other blankly. They telepathically asked each other, *'What is she talking about?'*

"I don't quite understand. Dr. Roe believes that Shannon will recover completely," Sue responded.

"We always hope that's the case, but right now, it looks like she's going to need at least a year of intensive speech, occupational and physical therapy. Frankly, we're not even sure she'll *ever* be able to hold a spoon by herself again. We'll do all we can, but..."

Sue's mind was racing:

...I don't believe what I'm hearing. They want to keep her for a year... in a broken down old TB hospital? They're going to teach her how to brush her teeth... to wash herself... to dress and eat without help? I can only visit for a couple of hours once or twice a week? They must be crazy. Shannon will never tolerate that kind of confinement... without her family and dog? No way! If she needs custodial care and retraining, *I'll be the one to do it*... I know her so much better than they do... they don't know what she really needs... do they really think I'll abandon my daughter to them? I can do it... but what happens after I die... who will take care of her then? ...

The conversation was relatively short and to the point. Sue felt like she was in the Twilight Zone. Melissa Anderson was polite and full of information, and had absolutely no idea how devastating her message had been.

This event provided another valuable lesson for us. I've always thought that people should believe *none of what they hear...and only half of what they actually see for themselves.* It's certainly a pertinent philosophy when applied to medicine.

Unfortunately, communication between health care workers is often flawed, and communication between caregiver and patient/family is not usually very effective. As a result, treatment regimen are often fallacious or at the least, inappropriate. Accordingly, it is incumbent on family members to gather and evaluate information for themselves, ask questions of caregivers, and participate in health care decisions. This was again one of those times.

Sue Eason and I met in Study Hall when we were in the tenth grade. We were fourteen years old, and were friends for many years before becoming engaged after our freshman year at the University of Georgia. What attracted me were her infectious smile, her intelligence, and her strength of will. Her heart and determination were much bigger than her five foot two inch frame.

In the four decades I had known Sue, I had never seen her be anything but calm when confronted with a problem or difficult situation. She was always strong, no matter how tough the challenge was. In fact, I've often said if I was caught in a major disaster, the person I'd most like to have with me is Sue. She is ever the problem-solver... and always without the slightest hint of panic.

The news she had just been given horrified her. When I arrived back at the hospital, she completely broke down for the first time in her life. Now it was my time to be the lifeline.

I told her not to worry about next week or next year. We would simply take each day as it came, and would do whatever we needed to do to make progress. I also promised to investigate rehabilitation options in Tennessee. In my heart, I just couldn't believe their prognosis was correct. I don't know if my optimism was misguided or appropriate, but I knew I wasn't yet ready to give in.

Wednesday afternoon brought another major upheaval. While the physical therapists had previously sat Shannon up briefly to test her strength, it was now time to get her on the edge of the bed and try to stand her up... if she could with a slight hip fracture. They then planned to move her to a chair to sit for a while. Not having supported her own weight for almost two weeks, she was very frail and unsteady. This would have been a difficult chore under the best of conditions, but having to cope with a combative brain injured patient made it almost impossible.

Laura and Cindi intended to move Shannon onto a backboard with straps on it, secure her tightly, and then turn the board upright so Shannon would be standing erect. Once she had some sense of balance, they would take the backboard away and use a walker to help her get to the chair. Shannon wanted no part of this exercise. She fought, screamed obscenities, cried, wiggled and just wouldn't cooperate with them. Why would she? She didn't have any idea what they were doing or why they were doing it.

Again, it was time for me to go into my 'I know the patient' mode. I took it upon myself to help get the process moving. I politely asked Laura to let me try to help. To the chagrin of everyone present, I leaned over Shannon, wrapped my arms under her arms and pulled her onto the backboard. Needless to say, she went ballistic!

Furthermore, when Shannon began to fight and scream, I just screamed back at her. Much to the horror of the nursing and therapy staff. It didn't faze the family, however, because they had seen us at odds over conditioning and training issues many times before.

It took a few minutes, but the mission was accomplished. Shannon was standing, and it was a pathetic sight. Her legs wobbled, her arms were strapped down, and she was dog-tired. In a few minutes we had her in a comfortable chair and under control again. She was finally at peace.

When it came time to move her back to the bed, she was very cooperative, and we were able to actually assist her in walking a few steps back to the bed. When she was settled back in the bed, she politely said, "Thank you." We were all astonished.

We learned another lesson during the exercise session. Stimulation is the best medicine for head injury victims. And it doesn't matter whether or not it's positive. Movement causes mental activity and forces the neurons to fire, activating the brain function. Shannon's ability to speak improved significantly for a while just after she was moved. We then saw alternating periods of humor, aggravation, frustration and apathy. It was all part of the normal course of brain injury recovery.

The day ended early, and Sue and Kim were set for *Hell Night* number two. Perhaps because they were mentally prepared for the worst, the night was slightly better. And so it went for the next ten nights... each one a little better than the one before.

Several friends and family members took turns on night duty: Richard and Sandra Eason; Lindsey and Cassie Clark; Martha Burks and her sister, Barbara; and Suzanne Eason, our 'niece-in-law' and practicing RN. Each person had some kind of unique experience they will remember for life. After the first week, however, it became possible for one person to handle Shannon at night. That task fell to Sue after Kelley and I returned to Murfreesboro the next week.

Thanksgiving day was pretty quiet; a little physical therapy, standing and walking between the chair and bed, and brief periods of talking. Much of the time, however, Shannon was just plain lethargic. The reason was that she was being given too much sedation through her IV. We finally called a halt to the medication, because we didn't think it was appropriate to slow down the mental processes of a brain injured patient trying to recover her faculties. Once the medication was discontinued, her awareness level improved dramatically. Had we not intervened again, who knows how long it would have taken her to regain her mental and physical balance?

The significant happening of the day came in the late afternoon. Lynn Crawford, our day nurse, assisted Shannon in brushing her teeth... an event that the Rehab Coordinator from Jerome Grant Hospital predicted would not occur for several months. We now knew that Shannon was *not* going to be transferred to the long-term rehab facility.

In contrast to the day before, Friday, November 24th was a very active day. A cystogram showed that Shannon's bladder was healing nicely and functioning normally. It signaled that the Foley catheter could be removed as soon as she was strong enough to safely walk back and forth from the bathroom. The occupational therapist also decided it was time to test Shannon's swallow reflex.

We were cautioned not to be overly distraught at Shannon's reaction when they put a spoonful of applesauce in her mouth. They told us that it was normal for her to gag... and spit the applesauce all over the room. In spite of the warning, we were very apprehensive. To everyone's surprise, however, she swallowed it with very little problem. Encouraged by her success, they gave her some orange juice. She swallowed it without incident. These two simple events justified our decision not to let the doctors insert the jejeunostomy tube. It would have been a mistake not to let her take food by mouth for several months.

By now, Shannon was capable of following most commands, and could assist us in moving her around in the bed, and from bed to chair. She had difficulty in sitting up in the chair for any length of time; she couldn't speak full sentences clearly; she couldn't hold a pencil well enough to write legibly; and still had several tubes and IVs in her.

She also looked ghastly. The combination of a partially shaved head; a stapled railroad track stretching from ear to ear; pock marked scabs on the side of her face from the shards of glass from the automobile window; and splotches of dried blood in her hair and around tubes, made her look like she was a creature out of a *Frankenstein* movie. Still, we had seen dramatic improvement in thirteen days. To us, she looked beautiful.

Samy and Jennifer returned to the watch on Friday afternoon, and were distressed by Shannon's appearance and lack of rudimentary physical skills. In spite of their anguish, they kept her company for the afternoon, alternately talking with her and reading while she slept. They were also fiercely protective if someone tried to disturb her.

During the next week, the staples were removed from Shannon's head and abdomen, and the drainage tube from her bladder. As she became more ambulatory, and could get to and from the bathroom with assistance, they also removed the Foley catheter and rectal tubes. Her physical, occupational and speech therapy became more intense... and often combative.

As the end of November approached, Shannon was capable of eating small amounts of food by mouth, although virtually all of her nutrition was gained through the G-tube in her stomach. Any real meals were still a couple of weeks away.

All in all, Shannon had progressed remarkably well physically... and now her mental status took center stage. At times, Shannon was cooperative and seemingly optimistic. At other times, she rambled incoherently about almost anything, and became upset and belligerent without warning. The slightest change in surroundings or people could alter her mood. She liked the nurses but intensely disliked the physical therapists. She liked Dr. Jenkins and Dr. Roe, but didn't like some of the others. It was during the third week after the accident that we realized there was a long and difficult gauntlet to be run, and much heartache to be experienced before this nightmare would, *if ever*, be over.

Shannon's traumatic brain injury (TBI) was defined as a 'nonhemorrahagic contusion in the left anterior temporal lobe and left inferior frontal lobe'. In plain English, she had sustained a tremendous blow to the left front of her skull, which severely bruised the brain. Fortunately, the injury did not result in any consequential bleeding or blood clots. That was good news because bleeding in the brain increases intracranial pressure, and typically results in either permanent loss of function or death.

So, two weeks after Shannon had awakened, it appeared that she was not going to be among the twenty-eight percent of brain injury victims who die from their injuries, nor the twenty-eight percent who require lifetime custodial care. The question was whether she was to be in the thirty-six percent of head trauma patients who suffer no long-term effects, or be among the eight percent who end up with some moderate disability. We were not to know the answer for many months.

As we arrived in room 616, we were bombarded with printed material explaining how the brain worked; possible effects of the trauma; the stages of improvement, recovery, and rehabilitation; and an extensive list of *do's* and *don'ts* of visitation. Throughout the two weeks Shannon was there, various para-professionals supplemented that information through intensive indoctrination about the inner workings of the brain as if they were preparing us for initiation into some kind of secret society. With no experience, and a great deal of naiveté, we were being ushered into the hidden world of brain disability.

Our instructions were clear. We were told to always remain calm; speak softly using simple words; call Shannon by her name often; tell her who we were; constantly tell her the day and time; give her plenty of time to respond to questions; correct her if she gave us a wrong answer... and above all, avoid arguments and stressful situations.

We were also told not to expect Shannon to understand much of what we said; not to ask her difficult questions; and not to expect her to remember who we were or any day-to-day activities. Further, we were cautioned not to use complicated words or words with double meanings; not to attempt humor; and not to talk down to her. Finally, they told us to avoid social talk with visitors in front of her.

We learned that the brain is actually very sensitive, and needs a great deal of protection. The skull provides the hard shell cover, and the cerebrospinal fluid that surrounds the brain provides the shock absorber that cushions the brain against bumps and blows.

We also learned about the brain stem, which controls the necessary functions of living. It determines consciousness, breathing, heart rate and, of course, swallowing. It also regulates messages to and from other parts of the body, and determines our reaction to heat, cold or pain stimuli.

Much of the early period was spent in trying to determine if there was any meaningful injury to the brain stem. Fortunately, it became clear within a few days that it had not been permanently damaged.

The neuropsychologist and psychosocial counselors explained to us that the trauma had caused damage to many brain cells, and we wouldn't know the extent of the damage until the swelling in the brain had decreased. They emphasized that Shannon may *improve* certain skills, but might not *recover* them completely. This, of course, was disconcerting because her future was just plain unpredictable. This air of uncertainty hung over Shannon, her friends, and family for more than four years.

We were instructed in the kinds of things we could do to hasten her recovery. The primary therapy was sensory stimulation. That involved doing or saying things to make Shannon become more aware of the world around her. We were warned that she would have periods of agitation, caused by the inner confusion of her brain cells. We were told that this agitation would manifest itself through such behaviors as shouting, cursing, hitting, kicking, or biting. All to the dismay of her family. While restraints are often needed to control patients when they become agitated, we opted to do this by human force. For Shannon and us, it was the best way.

Head trauma patients typically suffer some kind of memory loss. The type and extent of that loss depends upon which part of the brain is damaged, and how much brain cell destruction occurs. The severity and duration of the loss may not be known for an extended period of time.

Retrograde Amnesia refers to the loss of memory of people, places, events, or facts prior to the accident. The patient may lose a few minutes of time or virtually everything. Some or all of these bits of data may gradually return, or they may be lost forever.

Post Traumatic Amnesia begins just after the patient recovers consciousness. The patient cannot remember names or recite simple words or common facts because the brain is simply too confused. He or she is also unable to recall events that occurred just moments before. This is called short-term memory loss, and often lasts from a few days to a few weeks. Sometimes, however, it becomes a permanent impairment.

Perhaps the most debilitating type of memory loss is the *ability to learn* new things because it is a lifetime disability. Learning impairment may be manifested through either an inability to pay attention, speak, or store and recall information.

Three weeks after the automobile accident, we knew that Shannon had a good long-term memory, but we still had no way to assess whether or not she was suffering from Post Traumatic Amnesia or a permanent loss of her ability to learn.

From the day of Shannon's initial awakening on November 20th until she was discharged to a rehabilitation center on December 1st, we observed every classic behavior of a brain injured patient, and experienced the full gamut of emotions possible in the process.

Terror: It was a quiet Saturday morning and we wanted to give Shannon a sponge bath and comb her hair before any visitors began to arrive. That seemed easy enough. It only took a few strokes of the comb, however, to realize that her hair was such a mess of tangle and debris that it was an impossible task. Sue, Kelley and I reached the same conclusion almost immediately.

Since the front half of her head was already completely shaved, it only made sense to us that the remainder should be cut off too. It would be easier to manage for the next few weeks while she was regaining her ability to function independently. We also had to admit that she looked a bit frightful with no hair in front, a massive zipper scar in the middle, and a long flowing pony tail in the back.

Strangely enough, the floor nurses were not allowed to use a razor in the room, so hospital policy dictated that Shannon would have to be taken to the surgery suite to have the task performed. We thought putting her through a bureaucratic trip to the operating room was unnecessary, so we decided that we would cut her hair. After an hour or so of negotiations, we were able to 'borrow' some hair cutting shears from the operating room staff.

"Who's going to do it?" asked Sue.

"I guess, I am," I replied. "Kelley, I'm going to need your help to sit her up."

"Okay."

With that, I eased into the bed behind Shannon and sat her between my legs. So far, so good. Kelley faced Shannon, and talked to her as she braced her forward. As I started to shave her head, Shannon began screaming, grabbing and kicking.

"Daddy... Daddy... Daddy... *they're trying to kill me!* Help me, help me! They're killing me, *they're killing me!*" Shannon repeated that refrain at the top of her lungs for several minutes as she tried to jerk away. A simple job that should have taken less than a minute took us nearly ten minutes as we coped with her ranting and squirming. Once I turned off the shaver, Shannon immediately calmed down. She was so exhausted that she just lay back down, closed her eyes, and went to sleep.

Affability: Because of the infection that occurred at a needle site in the first few days after the accident, Dr. Jenkins had issued instructions to the nurses to change needle locations once every four or five days. It was a painful occasion for Shannon, as four IVs were pulled and relocated at a time.

"Shannon, it's time to re-position your IVs," the nurse said calmly. I'll be as careful as I can."

"Thank you," Shannon replied.

Then the grueling process began. It took probably fifteen minutes. Sue, Kelley and I winced each time Shannon was poked with a new needle. It didn't seem to bother her, however.

"Well... that should take care of us for a few days," the nurse said as she turned to leave.

"Thank you. Come back again sometime," retorted Shannon. Go figure.

Melancholy: During the last week at the Gwinnett Medical Center, Sue was Shannon's sole nighttime caretaker. She monitored her, groomed her, talked to her, and sometimes merely sat in the bed quietly with her arms around her.

Occasionally, during these intimate moments, Shannon appeared to have flashes of insight. While she could not yet speak clearly or consistently put words together correctly, Shannon was able to make her mother understand her feelings. Sometimes it was just the look in her eyes.

...Mom, I know something is wrong... but I don't know what. Why am I here? When can I go home? Am I going to get better? I'm trying...

"*I know*, honey... I know." In those moments, there was that special communication that only occurs between a mother and her child. An understanding that whatever the future holds, we'll do it together. It was that singular bond of unparalleled love between mother and daughter.

Apprehension: It was a Monday morning when the lively Trauma Coordinator, Kathy Dunbar, bounced into Room 616 with a wheelchair.

"Good morning, Shannon. How about a field trip? Would you like to take a spin around the hospital? It's such a nice morning, maybe we should go up to the patio on the roof and take a look. Would you like that?"

Shannon was undoubtedly bumfuzzled, but indicated agreement anyway. In a few seconds, Kathy, Sue and Shannon were on their way. As the door to the service elevator opened, Shannon began looking around as if she didn't know what was happening

It took less than thirty seconds to get to the top. The door opened, and Kathy pushed the wheelchair out to the helicopter pad where Shannon could look around and get some fresh air.

"I need to go back," Shannon uttered uneasily.

"You're doing fine, Shannon," Kathy reassured her.

I have to go back to my room now."

"Okay."

Thus ended the short outing. It was clear that the exposure to unfamiliar terrain had caused significant anxiety. Once back in the room, Shannon was much more comfortable.

Determination: It was around 11:00 p.m. on the last Wednesday night in Georgia. Shannon was restless, as she often was, and she wanted to get out of the hospital. She still had IVs in her arms, which were supported by a mobile IV pole; and, of course, the feeding tube in her stomach. By now she had enough strength to get up with help and move about the room. In other words, it took some force to restrain her.

"I gotta get out of here," she said as she flipped her legs off the side of the bed... with total disregard for any IVs or tubes.

"It's not time yet. Dad's coming back on Friday to

take us home to Tennessee. You have to be patient and get your rest."

Sue then grabbed Shannon's wrists and a titanic struggle began. For almost forty-five minutes, Shannon pushed and tugged trying to get out of bed. Sue countered mightily as the advantage shifted back and forth.

"I don't want to hurt you, Mom, but I gotta get out of here."

"Where are you going to go?"

"Home."

"Not tonight. We can go home in two days. Calm down and get back in bed. If you don't settle down, they're going to come in here and sedate you... and we'll *never* get out of here!"

At last the struggle was over.

Humor: Throughout the two weeks Shannon was in Room 616, we had a difficult time keeping her under the covers. Her fractured hip made her uncomfortable, and she continually moved up and down, and back and forth in the bed, throwing off the sheet, and exposing herself to the world.

"Shannon, if you don't keep yourself covered, we're going to have to charge all these guys twenty-five cents each," commanded her day nurse, Gerry, referring to the many male friends who had been to visit.

About an hour later, a young man accidentally walked into the room looking for another patient.

"That'll be twenty-five cents, please," Shannon ordered without hesitation. Sue and Gerry just looked at each other and laughed. It did signify something important, however. Shannon had at least some short-term memory.

These were just a few of the varied behaviors and emotions we observed and experienced. Little did we know that they were only brief indicators of the many things to come.

The last week was an exhausting one for Sue. While Kim and other family members sat with Shannon at various times during the day so Sue could eat, take a shower, or just get out of the hospital for awhile, by the end of the week Sue was just plain worn out.

As luck would have it, Rich and Suzanne, her nephew and 'niece-in-law', lived in a nice quiet neighborhood a couple of miles from the hospital. Throughout the ordeal they had offered their house as a refuge if Sue needed it. Finally, on Thursday she decided to take them up on their offer.

Sue arrived at the house around 2:00 p.m., hoping to get a couple of hours of sleep before returning for the last night at Gwinnett Medical Center. About thirty seconds after she put the key in the door, the alarm went off. Not having an access code, Sue immediately called her sister-in-law, Sandra, for instructions. Sandra gave her the code and she quickly turned off the alarm and went upstairs to the spare bedroom to lie down.

Sue had just closed her eyes when the doorbell rang. She slowly got up and went downstairs... puzzled as to who would be visiting in the middle of the day. It was the police. As soon as she opened the door she realized that they were responding to the alarm.

"Is this your house?

"No, it's my nephew's house."

"How did you get in?"

"I used a key they gave me." Sue then patiently explained all about the accident.

"Can you show us the key?"

"Yes." She produced the key and placed it in the lock to demonstrate her legitimacy. The police were finally satisfied. They got back in their car and sat for several minutes before leaving.

Sue went back upstairs, plopped down on the bed, and tried to go to sleep. It was no use. Embarrassed that she had disturbed the entire neighborhood, she just got up, washed her face, and went back to the hospital. She was as anxious to leave as Shannon. But that would have to wait until the next day.

---SIX---

The Military Operation

Friday, December 1, 1995, 7:47 a.m.

The drive from Murfreesboro to the airport in Smyrna, Tennessee took us just under half an hour, and I arrived full of anticipation. Today we were finally going to bring Shannon home.

Dr. George Eckles, our Clinic President and Shannon's new care coordinator, had picked me up at the Murfreesboro Municipal Airport where I had left my Jeep. The plan was to fly Shannon directly back to Murfreesboro, so the commute to the hospital would be safer and more convenient for her.

Dr. John Pearson was already there doing a final inspection of the airplane, and taking care of last minute paperwork for the one and a half hour flight to Lawrenceville, Georgia. Rick Smith, Sue's brother-in-law, was waiting for us at the airport in Georgia. Since the Gwinnett Medical Center was only two miles from the airport, we decided that it was appropriate to use Rick's van as a short-trip ambulance. Everything was set, and I was ready to roll.

The next thing I knew, we were down the runway and up in the air. It was a cool and sunny day, and the view was spectacular. We headed southeast above the wooded flat lands of East Tennessee, across the Appalachian Mountains, and over the rolling hills of North Georgia. I talked with John and George sporadically, but most of the time I was lost in reflection as I gazed at the last vestiges of yellow, brown and red leaves on the trees below:

...you know, during the last three weeks, we have certainly been blessed with the support of so many people... the physicians and staff of the Murfreesboro Medical

Clinic... the medical community... and so many business leaders... they have really demonstrated the true meaning of generosity and benevolence... at times it seems like virtually all 50,000 inhabitants have pitched in to help us in any way possible... everything from preparing meals for me, taking care of Haley, and keeping watch over the construction of our new house... it's been an emotional time... but it really helps to know that people *really* do care...

While Sue was back in Atlanta for the last week of November, I was busy trying to find a suitable rehab facility to temporarily house Shannon until we could occupy our new house. That was still three weeks away. In the eight months we had been in Murfreesboro, I hadn't realized there was a Center just across the street from our local hospital. Ironically, it was located in the original Murfreesboro Medical Clinic building.

Normally it took several weeks to get a patient admitted to the NHC Health Center. First, appropriate space had to be available; and often the Center was full. Second, the staff had to evaluate the patient's suitability for the facility and develop a daily care plan. Third, a Center standard called for a minimum stay of six months. Finally, there was the matter of economics. Shannon was not insured, and this usually causes disqualification.

Many of my Clinic physicians, as well as the hospital CEO, appealed on our behalf. As a result, management of the Center bent their rules and agreed to admit Shannon for up to a month... at a significantly reduced rate. Before she could be taken to the rehab center, however, she would have to be admitted to Middle Tennessee Medical Center for one or two days so she could be examined and tested to be sure she was medically stable. I was thinking:

...fate certainly smiled on us when Dr. Jenkins was on call the morning of the accident... not only has he taken

excellent care of Shannon, but how lucky was it that he and Dr. Eckles both trained at Emory?... without that connection, Dr. Jenkins would never have approved this high-risk transfer... we couldn't go by automobile because Shannon still needs constant medical supervision, and he doubts that she could tolerate a five-hour drive... the cost of ground or air ambulance transport is in the thousands of dollars... our only hope was a private plane... and here came Dr. Eckles to the rescue...

Dr. George Eckles is a general surgeon who completed his surgical residency at Emory University a few years before Dr. Jenkins. He left an excellent legacy, and when I told Dr. Jenkins that Dr. Eckles would be assuming the coordinator role for Shannon's transport and care, he readily agreed to the transfer.

Dr. Eckles is an imposing physical presence. He looks large... but his size belies his gentle manner, keen intellect, and precise surgical skill. He's a calm problem solver and true community servant, who's always looking for ways to make a positive contribution to society. One of those rare individuals in today's world who freely gives his time, energy and resources to others. A big man with a bigger heart.

In the week prior to the transfer, Dr. Eckles went about the task of talking to several physicians regarding participation in Shannon's care. Without exception, each agreed to do so...without charge. One of those physicians, Dr. John Pearson, was also a pilot. His aircraft was a little larger and could carry more weight than Dr. Eckles' plane, and he offered to take on the role of pilot for the mercy mission so Dr. Eckles could tend to Shannon if needed.

Without these two gracious men, Shannon would likely have remained in Georgia at Jerome Grant Rehabilitation Center, and the course of her recovery would surely have been much different.

❖❖❖

Rick and Kim Smith were waiting for us when we arrived in Lawrenceville a few minutes before 12:00 noon. Dr. Pearson remained at the airport to ready the plane for the return trip. Dr. Eckles and I jumped in the van, and we were off to the hospital.

The morning had not been a particularly good one for Shannon. Her occupational and physical therapy didn't go well, mostly because Shannon 'didn't feel like it'. Sue tried to spark some enthusiasm by continually reminding her that she was finally going to leave the hospital and go home to Tennessee. It didn't work. Shannon was now anxious about leaving familiar surroundings and heading into the unknown.

Dr. Eckles met with Dr. Jenkins to review the course of events since the accident, and signed some forms officially releasing Shannon into his care. This took no more than half an hour. All the while, we were gathering Shannon's belongings and loading them into the van.

Shannon was wearing... *what else*, a gray GEORGIA sweat suit, some tennis shoes, and a white SOUTH CAROLINA hat that Samy had brought her. The hat was to cover the gruesome surgical wound and her bald head. She could have cared less. Once again, this previously meticulous individual was completely unconcerned about her appearance. It was very painful to watch her indifference. Would she ever care again?

Several of the nurses, technicians and therapists came into Room 616 one last time to hug Shannon and wish her well. Many cried. Shannon was innately polite to each one, but didn't really understand what was happening. For all she knew, she was on her way to have another test or surgical procedure.

Now the real trouble began. We wheeled Shannon down to the van, she stood up, and we helped her into the seat.

"Where am I going?" she asked.

"Home to Tennessee," I said.

"Why?"

"So we can take care of you."

"Okay... *where?*"

"Don't worry about it. Dr. Eckles and Dr. Pearson are going to fly us home in Dr. Pearson's airplane. We're going to go to a new hospital for a couple of days, then to a rehabilitation center just across the street until the new house is ready."

"I don't want a new house. I like my apartment."

And so it went. What had been a promising week seemed to be ending with a whimper. It was later explained that too much new stimuli had overwhelmed her. Her mind couldn't find the right paths to assimilate all the changes happening at one time. In psychological terms, Shannon was 'flooding.' We were to learn much more about that phenomenon in the years ahead.

Rick was allowed to drive the van through the gate and directly up to the plane. Dr. Pearson was patiently waiting, and ready to depart at our command. We quickly loaded suitcases, gifts, and other paraphernalia into the storage bins in the wings, carefully balancing the weight on each side. In fifteen minutes we were ready to depart.

"Where are we going?" Shannon asked.

"Home to Tennessee," I responded.

"Why?"

"So we can take care of you."

"When can I go back to my room?"

"Honey, we're going to a new room in Tennessee."

"Okay."

It took us a few minutes to get situated in Dr. Pearson's six seat aircraft. There were two seats in the cockpit and four seats in the passenger cabin. Two seats were in single file along each side of the plane. We placed Shannon in the last seat so she could recline and sleep. Sue sat in front of her and I sat across from her.

"Okay honey, we need to put on your seat belt," I informed her.

"I don't want to," she replied.

"I'm sorry, but we have to."

As soon as I fastened the belt, she unfastened it. We repeated the sequence several times. Each time Shannon became more agitated. We finally relented. Against our better judgment, she didn't wear a seat belt.

We taxied down the runway and finally began our trek north. Somehow, the scenery didn't look quite as appealing. It was windy and the plane swayed back and forth, occasionally with a bump or dip. Ordinarily, this wouldn't have bothered us. But Shannon was annoyed. She complained, sometimes loudly.

"I want to lay down."

"Okay. I'll recline your seat." It wouldn't budge.

"Daddy... I want to lay down. *Now!*" It still wouldn't budge. We worked on it as we rocked back and forth. It was no use.

"Honey, just lie your head back, close your eyes and go to sleep. We'll be there in an hour or so."

"I want to get out. I don't want to stay here! *I've got to get out right now.*"

"I'm sorry. You'll just have to be patient. We'll be there soon." As if she could comprehend patience. If we hadn't realized how little memory or reasoning power Shannon had prior to this adventure... we certainly did now.

Dr. Eckles periodically asked us if we needed help. He even offered a sedative to calm her down. We refused because we didn't want to do anything to slow down her brain processes. I did strongly consider taking one of those pills myself, though!

Throughout the flight, Shannon alternately slid down in her seat, wiggled, or tried to get up. I could see the consternation in Dr. Eckles eyes. *'What have I gotten myself into'*, he must have been thinking. She complained about everything. It's too cold. It's too noisy. My hip hurts. You name it... and she complained about it. This was a new behavior that we were to see all too often in the weeks and months ahead.

It was after 2:00 p.m. when we sighted the Murfreesboro Municipal Airport. My first thought was:

...thank heavens... the ordeal is almost over...

My reaction was the same as it had been on the morning after *Hell Night*.

Kelley was waiting at the airport when we arrived. She hadn't seen her big sister in a week, and she was anxious to make up for lost time. While she could see definite improvement in Shannon, she too was disheartened by her complete disorientation to the world around her. Kelley struggled to fight back the tears.

Realizing that Shannon was under great duress, we carefully moved her from the airplane to my Jeep for the short trip to the hospital. In ten minutes we were at the front entrance to the Middle Tennessee Medical Center. We transferred her to a wheelchair and were allowed to take her directly to a room on the medical floor. Sue took care of the admissions paperwork.

By 3:00 p.m., the parade of doctors began. For the next several hours they poked and probed, and pronounced her fit for transfer the next day. Five of these physicians deserve special mention because of their prominence in Shannon's care, their long-term support and friendship... and their generosity. They did everything they could to help Shannon and us through the crisis and beyond, and took no payment for their services.

Dr. Warren McPherson is a Neurosurgeon who grew to be a good friend over the ensuing years. He has great charisma, and has been prominent in medical leadership throughout an illustrious career. I trusted him so much that he later operated on my back.

Dr. Dennis Bradburn was a Neurologist from our Clinic who played a major role in Shannon's life as she recovered. I say 'was', because Dr. Bradburn developed a particularly ravaging form of cancer in early 2000, and died only a few months later. At forty-four years of age. Such a tragic loss of a dedicated physician and friend.

Dr. Bob Ingle is a Gastroenterologist from our Clinic who tended to Shannon's nutritional needs and removed her G-Tube at the appropriate time. Dr. Ingle is always the consummate gentleman. Unassuming, calm, insightful and charitable, he's the true embodiment of the ideal physician.

Dr. Ray Lowery is an orthopedic surgeon who also became a long-term friend. He took care of Shannon's fractured collarbone and hip. Dr. Lowery is a physician who commands respect among peers and patients because he's intelligent, has terrific surgical skills, and most importantly, understands how to communicate with patients.

Dr. Tim Beasley was also once an Obstetrician/Gynecologist with the Murfreesboro Medical Clinic. He gave extraordinary support and encouragement to us over the next few months. While he is alive today, at age forty-nine he was severely injured in an automobile accident... ten months after Shannon's mishap. He is now unable to live independently, and is confined to a permanent domiciliary for the traumatic brain injured.

---SEVEN---

The Combat Zone

Saturday, December 2, 1995, 8:10 a.m.

Shannon had spent a restless night. She was in a strange place with an unfamiliar caregiver. Sue and I, on the other hand, had slept exceedingly well. It was our first night in the same bed in two weeks.

As plans for bringing Shannon home from Georgia began to take shape, the support staff of the Murfreesboro Medical Clinic had sprung into action. Departmental supervisors asked for volunteers to sit with Shannon in the hospital and rehab center so Sue, Kelley and I could have some time to take care of normal daily chores, tend to the final construction details on our house, and have the luxury of sleeping in our own bed for a few nights. Thankfully, there were at least two dozen of these prized co-workers.

Each individual consented to spend one night with Shannon or take two four-hour daytime shifts. This was of immense help because it allowed us to shed the blanket of fatigue that had overtaken us, and to regain a reasonable perspective on life. It was also quite an experience for many of them, as they witnessed Shannon's many mood swings, as well as her erratic and often irrational behavior. These individuals fulfilled a vital role because their interaction with Shannon provided very good therapy. Once again, the value of a support system was aptly demonstrated.

Dr. Bradburn completed the paperwork before Sue and I arrived, and we were allowed to take Shannon across the street to the NHC Health Center without delay. We wheeled her to my Jeep, helped her in, and drove around the block to the admissions entrance. Thank heavens she tolerated this change of scenery better than the previous day. The staff was prepared for us, and we were immediately taken to Room 151... Shannon's new home for the next two weeks.

Saturday was a cold and overcast day, and it foreshadowed the experience we would have in the rehabilitation center. Not because Shannon was treated poorly by the staff of nurses and therapists, but rather because of the nature of these kind of facilities.

Like many other domicilaries, NHC is a combination nursing home and rehabilitation facility. Many of the patients who arrive through the rehab path are eventually moved to the nursing home wing of the building. The sad fact is that it's extremely rare for anyone entering these facilities to ever recover enough function to live independently again. Accordingly, there is typically a pall of resignation and despair that permeates life here.

While we were thankful to have a place to house and treat Shannon for a couple of weeks, we quickly sensed the futility of the place as we accompanied Shannon to her room. We later learned that, at age twenty-four, she was the youngest patient in the Center by almost forty years.

Room 151 was somewhat more functional than Room 616 at the Gwinnett Medical Center. It looked like a hotel room---a microtel rather than a Marriott---but it did give us more room, drawer space, and a large toilet and shower area. This, of course, is important for access by the disabled.

While the room was equipped to accommodate two patients, the Administrator of NHC wanted to avoid housing an older patient with Shannon if at all possible. This turned out to be a blessing because Shannon's unpredictable behavior dictated that someone be with her at all times. I can only imagine the consequences of Shannon having a 'roommate'. The second bed was also a lifesaver for us personally.

While Shannon was still unsteady because she had been bed-ridden for three weeks, she was strong enough to walk with a walker. Throughout the afternoon, we would get her up and guide her through different areas of the Center so she could become acclimated to her surroundings. We hoped that this would lessen her anxiety and keep her calm. It did help somewhat, but we were still in for a nasty couple of weeks.

NHC had long, wide corridors with plenty of natural light from the outside. There was sufficient room for patients to either walk or be wheeled from place to place without obstructing visitors as they came and went throughout the day. It also left ample space for patients to be 'parked' outside their rooms in wheelchairs.

Some would greet visitors as they passed by, but others could only sit passively and watch the activity. Unfortunately, a majority of them were unresponsive patients, primarily stroke victims who had little chance of recovery. It seemed that their families had jettisoned them because home care was just not possible. It was a stark reminder of the ravages and ignominy of old age.

Before the end of the day we visited the recreation areas, Speech, Occupational and Physical Therapy Departments, and the cafeteria. While the cafeteria was actually quite nice, Shannon wanted no part of it. She simply didn't want to be treated 'like those old people'. She seemed most pleased with the physical therapy facilities, and was immediately ready for a 'workout'.

"I want to do my aerobics," she commanded.

"You're not quite ready yet, honey. You'll have to wait until Monday," I replied.

"Why can't I do them now?"

"There's nobody here to help you."

"I don't need help... I can do it myself!"

"Be patient for a couple of days."

"How long is that?"

The interchange continued for a couple of minutes until we diverted her attention to something else. Then we continued our rounds. At that point, two things were very clear. First, Shannon would recover her physical abilities long before her mental ones... and second, physical exercise would play a major role in the process.

Occupational therapy covers a broad scientific area designed to aid people in mastering their own environment. It encompasses everything from teaching individuals how to prevent workplace injuries to the rehabilitation of the sick or injured. The end point for every individual is the development of the skills necessary to master his or her own environment... whatever the scope of that environment. In the words of the American Occupational Therapy Association, 'occupational therapy is the job of everyday living'.

While much of the emphasis of occupational therapy has been centered on the workplace in recent years, it is still the more basic therapies that have the most profound effect on society. Most of us have some understanding of the need to teach workers how to prevent repetitive motion injuries, but few of us ever give a thought to teaching the ill or injured how to hold a comb, brush one's teeth, or take a shower. The focus of the occupational therapists at the NHC Health Center was on these rudimentary skills. Shannon had to master them before she could graduate to more advanced activities such as eating and drinking.

Physical Therapy encompasses the evaluation, treatment and prevention of physical disability and/or pain associated with virtually any injury, disease, or disability. Therapeutic interventions involve the use of manual manipulation or support, mechanical devices, or electrical stimulation that aid in improving posture, locomotion, strength, endurance, cardiopulmonary function, joint mobility, flexibility and overall coordination. The intended end result is a healthy body with maximum functional abilities.

For Shannon, it meant movement and exercise. Because these activities had played such a prominent role in her young life, she enjoyed the physical challenges and quickly outperformed the standards set for her by the PT staff at NHC. In a matter of two weeks, she recovered a substantial amount of her strength and endurance. Her only major physical deficit was the lack of flexibility, which was hampered by her fractured hip and clavicle, and her ten-inch abdominal incision. It was well over a year before Shannon could bend and stretch again anywhere near her pre-accident levels.

Speech Therapy involves the treatment of any malady that affects an individual's ability to hear the spoken word, comprehend language, or speak in a coherent manner. Speech therapists also deal with swallowing disorders. The field covers a wide variety of disorders or irregularities including Autism, stuttering, Dyslexia, accents, post larynx surgery rehabilitation, and aphasia/dysphasia.

Dysphasia is a milder form of the more commonly known affliction called aphasia... an impairment of the ability to use or comprehend words. Typically these ailments are the result of head injuries or strokes, and it was the primary area of concentration in Shannon's treatment at NHC. At the time, we didn't know whether she was suffering from dysphasia or aphasia. If it was the former, we had a much better chance of full or near full recovery. If it was the latter, life was going to be much more difficult for Shannon.

Weekends are usually long periods of inactivity for patients confined to rehabilitation facilities. There is no therapy, and only a skeleton staff of nurses. It is simply a time of bare maintenance, or at least it was for Shannon. On this first weekend, we tried to watch television, talk to Shannon, and play simple word games. She was not happy.

Two of our Clinic staff members stayed with Shannon on Saturday and Sunday nights. Sue, Kelley or I remained until Shannon was asleep and then turned the watch over to one of them.

On Saturday night, Shannon was disoriented and agitated, and made life difficult for her caregiver, Fran Trumbull. She was more than a hand full as she became belligerent and threatening. It was *Hell Night* all over again, and Fran was the victim. Unfortunately, she was just too mild mannered to handle a strong-willed, irrational tempest. The look of relief on her face when we arrived on Sunday morning told the whole story.

The second night was not as bad, or perhaps our caregiver, Nancy Warren, was just better prepared for what was to come. Nancy was our Urology Department Manager, and the daughter of a physician. Nancy is every bit as strong-willed as Shannon, and it appears that she applied her considerable diplomatic and leadership skills to coax and cajole Shannon into obeying orders. They spent a great deal of that night wandering the hallways of the Center.

Because Shannon was so difficult to handle those first two nights, many of the original caregiver volunteers decided to opt out of nighttime duty. Who could blame them? She was our daughter, but even *we* became wary because it was a constant battle to keep her contained. A few individuals did watch her during the day for the next two weeks, which was a great relief for us.

A treasured member of the family was our dog,

Haley. No matter what problems befell any one of us, Haley was our refuge. While Brian, Shannon and Kelley no longer lived at home, the first thing they did when they visited was look for her. The stroke of her black and white hair always made them feel truly at home... comfortable and serene.

Shannon and Kelley always volunteered to keep Haley when we traveled, and sometimes they would drive hundreds of miles to make the transfer. Now that Shannon was in Murfreesboro, we were convinced that the best therapy we could provide was a visit with her pet. For several days prior to the relocation from Georgia, we told Shannon that she was going to Tennessee to see Haley. Finally, on Sunday afternoon, the much-awaited visit was to take place.

It was another blustery day with snow flurries. Sue put a coat and hat on Shannon and took her outside to the courtyard while I parked the car and put Haley on the leash. When we got within a hundred feet of Sue and Shannon, Haley's tail began wagging energetically, and she pulled me toward her family members.

"Who is that?" Shannon asked earnestly.

"It's Haley," I replied somewhat taken aback.

"Oh."

Sue and I were distressed. We watched as Shannon had only a passing interest in her own dog! She stroked her head gently, as if she were petting a neighborhood stray, and then promptly wanted to go inside. The visit lasted ten minutes.

Our spirits were lifted somewhat later in the day, however, when Shannon insisted on taking a shower. Sue got in with her and showed her what to do. Shannon's first meaningful shower in almost a month clearly improved her disposition... for the time being.

❖❖❖

Monday was evaluation day. Sue and Shannon first met with the Speech Therapy Director, who indicated that she would draw up a plan for the week. The first session would be on Tuesday. Then they talked with staff members in the Occupational Therapy Department. Since Shannon could now take care of her basic grooming needs, they decided to skip 'Life Skills 101' and move her on to the advanced course; cutting and pasting, making simple jewelry, and baking cookies in a toaster oven.

The upheaval of the day came in Shannon's favorite venue. She was scheduled for her first physical therapy session in the early afternoon. Much to her dismay, it was a group session with approximately fifteen elderly stroke victims, all sitting in a circle. Sue and Kelley attended with her.

"Mom, this doesn't look good," Kelley observed.

"I know. We'll just have to bear with it and see what happens," Sue replied warily.

"I don't want to be here," Shannon announced to the class.

Most of the patients were in a wheelchair, including Shannon. Before the instructor could begin, all eyes turned to Shannon, and she wasn't amused.

"Good afternoon, everyone. How's everybody doing today? Let's start by having each of you tell us your name and where you live."

Some patients joyfully complied, while others could barely hold their head up, much less talk. Each patient responded as best they could until they got to Shannon, who was very hesitant. Eventually, she was able to mumble her name, but she didn't know where she lived.

"I'm Shannon's mother. Shannon lived in Atlanta until she was in an automobile accident a few weeks ago, and will now be living with us in Murfreesboro."

Shannon looked back at Kelley and said, "Kelley, I need to go now."

Kelley was just as anxious to get out of the room as Shannon, but told her sister to be patient for a few more minutes.

The 'workout' consisted of hand exercises such as clapping and patty-cake movements in different sequences. Then they handed a softball sized rubber ball from person to person around the circle. Even in her limited mental state, Shannon felt demeaned by the process.

After the session, Sue talked with the instructor, and it was readily agreed that Shannon was out of place in the class. From then on, she was given individual instruction with much more advanced exercises on a stair-stepper and treadmill.

Shortly after returning to Room 151, things began to brighten. Dr. Bradburn came in to see Shannon, and he was pleased with her progress. He was ready to transition her to solid food, and left orders to begin with small meals three times a day. Depending upon how much she was able to eat, she would continue to receive supplements through the G-Tube in her stomach.

Dr. Bradburn was astute enough to recognize that Shannon was uncomfortable being held captive in a domiciliary designed for older patients, and needed more stimulation.

"Dennis, the sun is out and the temperatures have warmed into the mid fifties, is it possible for us to take Shannon out for a ride or something?" I quizzed Dr. Bradburn.

"That just might be the ticket," he replied. "It's a little unusual at this stage, but I think it's a good idea. I'll write an order. Just don't overdo it, and have her back here before dark. Depending on the weather and how she feels, maybe it would be a good idea to get her our each day for a while."

Even though Shannon had significant difficulty in assimilating words and ideas, she clearly understood the concept of freedom. Immediately after Dr. Bradburn gave us the okay, Shannon got up from the chair and reached for her jacket. At 3:00 p.m. we were in my Jeep and on our way for a tour of town and a visit to our nearly completed new house.

The two-hour excursion was excellent therapy. Shannon was much more alert than she had been three days earlier when we flew her up from Georgia. She showed more interest in the world around her, and even commented occasionally on the way some houses looked, the bareness of the trees, and other elements of the environment that most of us take for granted.

Complacency and the absence of emotion are two serious, and relatively common, consequences of brain injuries. The patient simply shows no interest in people, pets, events or activity. Our short trip gave us encouragement that Shannon was regaining some of her personality. We were also pleased that she began to complain about the pain in her shoulder and hip. This, we thought, was good. In later weeks, however, we weren't so pleased because we couldn't stop her complaining.

Sue stayed with Shannon on Monday night. For the most part, it was a calm and restful one, and they both managed to get a fair amount of sleep. As we look back now, it makes perfect sense that Shannon would feel more secure with her mother present than with strangers... even if they were well-meaning friends. We were certainly not through with Shannon's moodiness, aggression, anger or fear, but the night of December 4th was definitely a turning point.

Tuesday was the first day of boot camp. First, a shower, a good teeth brushing, and a change of clothes. Then breakfast. A full can of ENSURE through the feeding tube. Next was Occupational Therapy, where the staff worked on Shannon's fine motor movements.

Lunch was a major event, however. Just after noon the nurse brought in a tray of mashed potatoes, green beans and chocolate milk. Shannon dived into the food like she hadn't eaten in a month... which, of course, she hadn't. Sue continually cautioned her not to eat too much, too fast. After so much apprehension about Shannon's swallow reflex, our fears were finally put to rest. It was now just a matter of time before the PEG could be removed.

The afternoon physical therapy session was very taxing. Shannon walked on the treadmill and stair-stepper for five to ten minutes. True to her personality, she pushed herself too much, and was totally exhausted when she arrived back in Room 151. It was just as well, however, because it was too cold and rainy to take an afternoon ride.

Sue and I were relieved for dinner by another one of our caregiver friends. In the hour and a half we were gone, Shannon created havoc. She didn't like being 'watched' by a stranger, and wanted to 'check out of this place'. She was angry, loud and abusive, forcing the nurse to sedate her. We were not pleased. Once again, in the eyes of the nursing staff, the only solution to her disruption was medication.

The next two days were merely maintenance days. Therapy sessions were not very productive, and Shannon seemed to lack energy and enthusiasm. The only positive development was the complete discontinuance of her tube feedings. All nourishment was now being taken by mouth.

Once again, our earlier observation about medication proved to be correct. Invariably, Shannon would have a hangover for two days after being sedated, and she was so lethargic that therapy of any kind was essentially a waste of time. She seemed to regress for a few days until we could re-energize her. Accordingly, we never let them sedate her again.

We picked up the pace on Friday. I arrived at NHC around 7:30 a.m. to give Sue a breather so she could go to our apartment, eat breakfast, and take care of some personal chores.

After Shannon completed her morning shower and grooming, I shaved her legs. It was a ritual that began while she was still semi-conscious a few weeks earlier, and continued because Shannon was still not cleared to handle a razor. Why me? Because Sue often nicked her legs in the process, and I never did. Then it was on to breakfast; oatmeal and, of all things, *skim milk*. Here was a severely underweight, hollow-looking patient who steadfastly refused to drink whole milk.

Speech therapy was very promising. Shannon showed signs that she was starting to remember things that had happened only a few hours ago. Recovery of her short-term memory was an indication that she was suffering from dysphasia, not the more malignant memory disorder, aphasia. This again raised our hopes for a near full recovery.

Sue was impressed with Shannon's recall of historical events. With some prompting from the therapist, Shannon was able to correctly regurgitate a few dates, events, and famous people. She had more difficulty with recent history, however, and could not easily remember the President of the United States.

Her inability to articulate answers promptly created frustration for her because she knew the answers but couldn't always find a pathway through the brain to her speech center. This is a common occurrence in brain injuries, and it persists in Shannon even today...although certainly not to the same extent.

Her 'homework' assignment was to create a Memory Book to record daily events and current happenings. The purpose was to stimulate her thought processes and begin to rebuild her personal history. We later found the Memory Book to be a very important tool in her emotional recovery because she eventually became obsessed with recapturing her lost months of memory. In the process, we learned how worrisome and debilitating amnesia can be.

Shannon had a very good day in physical therapy. She did some aerobics, walked on the treadmill, and successfully completed several coordination exercises involving a beanbag. In the process, however, she developed a headache. She was given a Tylenol tablet by mouth, which solved the problem. This may not seem to be a particularly important event in the overall picture, but in actuality, it was very promising sign.

We were told that most brain-injury patients suffer from severe headaches for years after the trauma, and that over-the-counter medications rarely relieve the pain. Once she was feeling better, she was ready for her afternoon outing. Sue took her to the apartment to see Haley, and this time she was much more responsive. Haley lifted her spirits considerably, although Shannon now began exhibiting signs of depression. We deduced that from the fact that she began 'ragging' on herself with regularity.

"Mom, I'm a GROSS MESS," Shannon said as she looked in the bathroom mirror.

"No you're not. In time, the wounds will heal, your hair will grow out, and once again you'll have a beautiful face."

"I'm weak and skinny, and I look awful. I'm going to be ugly forever!"

"Don't be too hard on yourself. Give it some time, and you'll see that I'm right. In a month or two, you'll look just like you used to."

"These braces hurt, and they keep cutting my mouth. My hip hurts. My shoulder hurts. I'm tired."

"You'll be okay. You just have to be patient."

Thus began a new pattern of behavior. For the next

several months, Shannon complained incessantly about everything animal, vegetable or mineral. If she saw it, heard it or felt it... she complained about it. But in the grand scheme of things, the experts told us that complaining was much better than apathy. While it was difficult to bear at times, we took them at their word.

That night, Sue and I were scheduled to attend the Clinic Christmas Party at the Stones River Country Club. We were looking forward to getting away for a few hours, and Kelley volunteered to stay with Shannon for the night. It was a nice thought... but it just wasn't to be. The night was destined to be a rough one.

Dinner was late and the nurse was insensitive, so Shannon took out her frustration on Kelley.

"I don't like her. I'm not hungry and I'm *not* eating! I want to leave. I'm going to leave and *you're* staying here," Shannon said in disgust.

"No you're not. You're not going anywhere, and neither am I," Kelley replied.

"I don't want to eat. I want to get out of here!"

"We can't. Mom and Dad would be *real* angry if we did that."

Shannon had no intention of listening to Kelley. Under normal circumstances, she would respect authority, but this was her *little* sister... and Shannon wasn't about to obey commands from her. The use of surrogate authority might work, however. So, in an effort to get results and keep the peace at the Center, Kelley constantly reminded her that Mom and Dad would not be happy if she ignored their requests. In Kelley's eyes, it was the only way to get her cooperation.

Shannon then abruptly got out of bed and started packing clothes in a suitcase. Kelley tried to stop her... and that was a big mistake. Shannon was now in full fury, and was ready to battle anyone in her way. Kelley tried to calm her so the nurse wouldn't have to sedate her again. The more she tried, the more unreasonable Shannon became.

"Get out of my way. I'm checking out!"

"Shannon, please just get back in bed before the nurse comes in here and gives you a shot."

"Just let her try. I'll punch her lights out!"

As Kelley was trying to gently restrain her, Shannon grabbed her sister and literally threw her against the wall with enough force to move the table by the bed and knock it's contents onto the floor. It should be noted that Shannon was 5'3" and 110 pounds at the time. Kelley was 5'8" and outweighed her sister by more than thirty pounds.

"Get out of my way. I'm leaving here... and I want a knife."

As she started toward the door, Kelley pushed her in the direction of the bed and held her arms so she wouldn't pull the tube out of her stomach. They wrestled around on the bed for a couple of minutes before Shannon was finally subdued.

Once she was calm, Kelley went into the bathroom to get a washcloth to wipe the sweat off of Shannon. While her back was turned, Shannon walked past her into the hall and made a beeline for the nurses' station.

"I'm Shannon Lloyd in Room 151. I want a knife."

The two nurses just looked at each other.

"I need a knife and I need one *now*!"

The nurses didn't really know how to react because they had no experience with a young brain-injured patient. Here came Kelley to the rescue.

"I'm sorry for the disturbance. She's my sister, and she does *NOT* need a knife. She just doesn't like this tube in her stomach. I'll take care of her."

Kelley then tried to lead Shannon back to her room, but this didn't go smoothly. Shannon broke out of Kelley's grasp and headed for her neighboring patient's room.

"Excuse me…" she called to her neighbor as Kelley grabbed her around the waist and pushed her back toward her room.

"Kelley, I want to go home. I'm calling Dad."

"No, you're not. I'm responsible for you tonight and I'll be really upset if we ruin their one night to rest and have some fun. Besides, you don't know their telephone number."

"Yes, I do."

"No, you don't," Kelley responded as she unhooked the telephone cord from the wall while Shannon was getting into the bed.

"I'm going to see if they'll heat up your food. You need to eat now. It will make you feel a hundred times better, I promise. Maybe I can get you some chocolate, too. You just hang tight, I won't be a minute."

Kelley headed out to the nurses station with one eye on the door. Whereupon, Shannon plugged in the telephone cord, picked up the receiver, dialed '9' to get an outside line, and carefully dialed the telephone number to our apartment that was written on the grease board on the wall opposite the bed.

Sue and I were dressed for the party and were just about to leave when the telephone rang.

"Hello." There was a brief silence as Kelley grabbed the phone from Shannon's hand.

"Dad? … it's Kelley."

"Is everything okay?"

"Yes, everything's fine. I just wanted to tell you to have a good time."

I could now hear Shannon in the background, and I knew there was trouble. It took a few minutes to pry the story out of Kelley because she didn't want to spoil the evening. I was now irritated, and told her I was on the way. I quickly changed clothes, and left Sue and Haley for the night.

As I hung up the telephone, I thought to myself:

...here we go again... when is this ever going to end? ... I've had enough... I'll take care of this behavior problem tonight once and for all...

There is much truth to the adage that 'it's always darkest before the dawn'. I arrived at Room 151 about 8:00 p.m., and really let Shannon have a piece of my mind. According to the brain injury experts, confronting Shannon was the wrong thing to do. These specialists insist that it was not likely that she understood a word of what I was saying, and probably even became more confused.

They may very well be right, but the proof is in the results. Shannon readily obeyed all of my commands, ate some of her cold dinner, and got in bed quietly. She was still somewhat restless and wanted to get out of the rehab center, but I made it plain to her that she was going to be there for another week, so she had better make the best of it.

While her sister knew it wasn't the real Shannon talking during these times, it was still difficult for Kelley to be the recipient of such bad treatment. Kelley had been an enormous help to Shannon, and it was difficult for her to juggle school, work, and her own emotions while trying desperately to coach her sister back to health. There is no doubt, however, that the close relationship between these two siblings played a critical role in Shannon's recovery.

After midnight, Kelley and I got in to the spare bed and slept... or attempted to sleep, for the remainder of the night. Shannon rested very peacefully. Somehow we had avoided *Hell Night* number three.

Saturday was a much better day. We loaded a chair, table and portable TV into the Jeep and took Shannon over to our new house while Sue and I did some cleaning. Shannon liked the house, and seemed to generate some real enthusiasm for moving the next weekend. We were pleased to see her excited about it.

All in all, Shannon enjoyed her day out. She ate well, and reluctantly went back to the Center in the late afternoon. She complained about her feeding tube, and her other aches and pains, but she also expressed satisfaction several times during the day. We felt that we were now making meaningful progress.

Sunday was another active day. After our morning grooming ritual, we left NHC and went to spend the day at our small apartment. Shannon was slightly depressed, probably because she was starting to understand her situation a little better. Sue constantly tried to reassure her, but confessed to me confidentially that she'd probably be just as bewildered and angry if she were in the same situation.

Haley had been left alone a great deal of the time for the past five weeks, and was really happy to have the company of her family and Kelley's roommates for several hours. Shannon helped Sue do some packing, but seemed to tire very quickly. Sue attributed this to boredom mixed with depression.

Around noon, we received a telephone call from Doctors Dorothy and Wayne Murphy, who wanted to bring us some lunch. They came by for a brief visit and left us a veritable feast. Needless to say, we ate very well for the next couple of days. The day passed quickly, and finally it was time to return to NHC. Shannon didn't want to go, but we reminded her that she needed a few more days of therapy before she could come home for good.

Because of the several hairline fractures in Shannon's jaw, Dr. Tom Leonare had installed 'arch bars' on Shannon's teeth during his full facial makeover on November 15th. These arch bars were nothing more than industrial strength braces, which were mounted *in* the gums, not *on* the teeth. Needless to say, they were painful and irritating, and drove Shannon to distraction.

Their purpose was to hold the jawbones together while the jaw mended. The price paid by the patient was high, however. It was not only difficult to chew, but any misstep caused gashes in various places in the mouth. So, along with the more major problems, Shannon had to contend with a sore mouth for almost two months.

Soon after we returned to Room 151, we had a visit from Dr. Alex Hollis, an Oral & Maxillofacial Surgeon. He had been asked by Dr. Eckles to look at Shannon's fractured jaw and evaluate her bite. He found that she was developing an under bite because the lower part of the jaw was beginning to protrude as it healed.

Dr. Hollis gave us two alternatives for solving the problem. It could be repaired surgically, or by putting some small, but powerful, rubber bands on the braces to bring her jaw together and correct the bite. We decided to try the non-surgical solution first. Fortunately, this simple approach eventually corrected the problem... but not without much discomfort along the way.

By Monday, December 11th, we had decided that Shannon needed to get out of the rehab center as quickly as possible because she was now outpacing all forms of therapy... and was increasingly frustrated with 'being in an old people's jail'. Before we could leave, however, the G-Tube had to be removed from her stomach, and Dr. Bradburn had to give his permission.

I made arrangements for Dr. Ingle to remove the tube on Wednesday in the SurgiCenter of the Murfreesboro Medical Clinic, even though I was scheduled to be in Washington, D.C. representing the Medical Group Management Association before the Physician Payment

Review Commission. Once again, Sue was left as the sole caregiver. I knew Dr. Ingle would take good care of Shannon, but I really hated not being there to give her comfort and support.

Monday and Tuesday were uneventful, routine days. Shannon was gaining strength daily, although she was still considerably under weight. Occupational therapy had ceased, and the emphasis was shifted to speech therapy. Her speech therapists, Beth and Jennifer, were delighted at Shannon's progress in memory and recall of facts. Shannon was not. She was angry that she had to be re-taught things she already learned in school.

"Shannon, you're doing great. Just be patient. In a few months, all of those things locked up in your head will resurface... I promise you. Don't be so hard on yourself."

"Mom, I'm just stupid," Shannon replied intensely.

"We'll just keep working on it until we get there, okay?"

"Okay."

For the rest of the week, Sue and Shannon worked on her Memory Book and took day trips to keep from becoming bored.

Shannon's feeding tube was removed early on Wednesday morning under a mild anesthesia. Predictably, she was sluggish for the next two days. Nonetheless, when I arrived back in Room 151 on Thursday night, I was amazed at how much progress Shannon had made in three days. Except for having some difficulty putting words together at times, she seemed much more like her old self. Medically, Shannon was ready to move on. Mentally, there were still many challenges ahead.

Needless to say, the staff at NHC was dismayed that we planned to take Shannon home on Saturday. They tried to convince Sue that she needed many more weeks of supervision and therapy. Sue was tactful, but firm, in explaining to them that we had the capacity to properly supervise her... and would certainly pursue appropriate outpatient therapy. Dr. Bradburn gave his approval, and Shannon was released from the Center on December 16th. She felt as though she had been sprung from prison.

As we look back on Shannon's thirty-six days of confinement, it seems much longer. It was certainly the most intense period of our lives. We were confronted with tragic news, and given very little hope for her survival. We went through alternating periods of optimism and despair as she made progress, only to regress again.

In the darkest hours, we went through a lot of soul searching... and prayed that Shannon would survive and be able to live a normal life. Admittedly, however, there were times when we had doubts about what was best for her. We could only hope God would guide us in the right direction.

We experienced the best and the not-quite-so-good in the Health Care System. We found emergency personnel, doctors, nurses and therapists who displayed skill, kindness and insight as they tended to Shannon's medical and custodial needs. We saw others who were cold, clinical and by-the-book practitioners. To some, Shannon was just another interesting 'case' in their daily routines; to others she was a valuable young woman with much to live for. We were thankful that the vast majority seemed to truly care about Shannon as a person.

We also learned that the best-intentioned caregivers don't always have the answers. They make decisions and give advice based on their education, experience, and biases. The major flaw in their approach is that they typically don't really know the patient. This is why it's absolutely critical for family and friends to play an active role in decision-making and development of treatment regimens.

Our experience confirmed that a proper balance of trained experts and insightful family make a powerful combination in patient care. There were at least four times when our intervention in the care process avoided what could have been serious errors in those first thirty-six days; any one of which would undoubtedly have resulted in a much different outcome.

As we left the Center on that beautiful Saturday morning, I thought of Winston Churchill's famous observation as the tide of World War II was turning in the fall of 1942:

'This is not the end. It is not even the beginning of the end. But it is, perhaps, the end of the beginning'. How prophetic those words proved to be.

---EIGHT---

The Return of Hope

Saturday, December 16, 1995, 6:15 p.m.

It had been a long but rewarding day. We managed to spring Shannon from Room 151 at the NHC Health Center, and move furniture from two different locations into our new home. We had lots of help in the process, and in some ways, the day was almost festive.

For the first time in quite a while, we had Brian, Shannon and Kelley together, along with Shannon's steadfast friends, Jennifer and Kim, and my brother, Ken. Each of us took turns entertaining Shannon while the others carried boxes, moved furniture, and performed routine clean-up chores. At the end of the day we were more optimistic about the future.

Shannon tolerated the chaos extremely well, and at times seemed almost normal. In reality, however, she was performing by rote, and clearly had little understanding of what was happening. Throughout the day she said things to Jenn and Kim that led us to believe she thought she was back in her sorority house at the University of Georgia. That didn't matter to us. We were just happy to have her home.

The next forty-three days were full of positive events, although they were not without some significant challenges. The initial dilemma came on our first night home.

While Shannon no longer had a tube in her stomach, we still had an uneasy feeling about her outbursts of anger, confusion, and fetish with knives. Frankly, we didn't know what she might do in the middle of the night if she woke up and began roaming around a new house. Accordingly, we collected every knife and sharp instrument we could find and put them in a safe place so we could rest easily. After a couple of uneventful nights, we concluded that our worries were unfounded, and we restored all potential weapons to their rightful places.

Brain injury experts stress that it is important for patients to stay busy and involved. Stimulation of any kind causes the electrical activity in the brain to increase, facilitating neuron-to-neuron communication. When these nerve cells are activated, they carry messages along a 'chain' of millions of neurons, enabling us to execute all the functions of daily living. Just like lifting weights or playing the piano, the more one trains, the better one performs. Accordingly, we made every effort to keep Shannon active and engaged so her ability to recall, think and reason would be enhanced.

Our first two weeks home were during the holiday season, and we had lots of visitors and much activity. It was then that we also learned that *too* much diverse activity could be detrimental. Just as excessive weight lifting can cause overuse injuries, Shannon's attempts to talk too much overloaded her injured neuron chain.

When Shannon first began to speak after awakening from her coma, she experienced difficulty in formulating her words and putting together coherent sentences. It seemed to us that the problem was getting better with each passing day. However, the combination of visits from her friends, family, and my co-workers, coupled with the holiday activities, bewildered Shannon. Often a sentence intended to say:

"My hip hurts when I stand too long," turned out like this:

"My hurt hips when I long too stand." This impairment is known as dysnomia. It is simply the inability to select or retrieve the correct word, and is exacerbated when the patient is forced to access his or her vocabulary faster than he or she can process the information. It most often happens in group conversation or a fast paced environment. Once Dr. Bradburn explained what was happening, we did a better job of controlling the amount of stimulation, thus improving the problem dramatically within a few days.

A couple of days before Christmas, Samy made the trek from Columbia, South Carolina to Murfreesboro to add some spice to our lives. He followed directions perfectly, and showed up at our house just after noon on Tuesday.

"What's for lunch?" he quizzed, as he emerged unannounced into the kitchen.

"Samy, you almost scared the life out of me," retorted Sue.

"And how is our patient today?"

"See for yourself." Whereupon they walked into the family room where Shannon was sorting pictures she had unpacked from a box.

Samy was really pleased with what he saw. Shannon was now up and active all day, except for an occasional nap. The last time Samy had seen her, she was essentially bed-ridden. It only took a minute for them to hug and start jabbering like the old friends they were. If Samy was dismayed by Shannon's inability to articulate correctly, he never let on.

It wasn't long before Samy also gained some first-hand experience with Shannon's unpredictability. Prior to moving, we ordered a satellite dish from a local outlet so we could have nightly entertainment and, of course, the college football bowl games. The installer showed up in mid-afternoon.

"Who is he... and what does he want?" Shannon asked angrily.

"He's here to install the satellite dish so we can watch television," Samy replied.

"I don't like him. He's a spy. He wants to rob us. Get him out of here!"

"It's okay. He's not a spy, and he's here to help us. Let's go in your room and look at some pictures."

"I don't trust him. We have to stay here and watch him so he doesn't steal something!"

"He's not going to take anything. He's just going to put in some wires and a dish."

This exchange went on for a few minutes as Samy and Sue searched for a way to calm Shannon. Finally, they went into her room and looked at photographs of their college days, and her agitation disappeared as quickly as it came. Unfortunately, that wasn't the end of the story.

An hour or so later, the installer was ready to drill a hole in the floor to run the cable up from the crawl space into the family room. Shannon pronounced that he was incompetent, and that she could do a better job. In her mind, he was destroying the structural integrity of the house. Except for brief times of diversion, Shannon railed against the intruder for the entire afternoon and much of the evening. Trying to reason with her was useless, and it was quite a chore just containing her. By the next day, the episode was forgotten, at least by Shannon.

The next evening provided one of the most unnerving, but hilarious, moments we experienced during the entire recovery period. It was shortly after dinner when Shannon was strolling around the bay window in the kitchen. Without warning, she began to hallucinate.

"Mom... *Mom*, there's a giant rabbit eating the trees in the front yard!"

"What?" replied a startled Sue.

"You better do something quickly, before he eats them all. Hurry!"

Sue went to the window and looked at the row of

newly planted trees approximately two hundred feet from the house. There was ample moonlight, but she didn't see a thing. By now, we were all carefully examining the landscape through the window... and looking at each other for any indication that anyone understood what Shannon was seeing. Everyone was perplexed because there was no evidence of any activity in the yard.

"Don't worry, honey, the rabbit's gone now. Everything is fine."

"No, Mom... he's still there. *Look*! If you don't go out and get him, I will."

Sue grabbed the flashlight, quickly made her way out the side door, and headed for the trees. What she found was a squirrel scampering around several feet in front of the trees. Periodically, he would rise up on his hind legs as if he were looking for something.

Then she saw it. Because of the position of the squirrel and the angle of the moonlight, there was a sizeable shadow that, indeed, looked like a rabbit. Sue could only chuckle. She chased the squirrel away and became the hero of the day.

We were careful not to express amusement in Shannon's presence because she would have been offended. Later, Sue, Samy and I did have a great laugh, however. Actually, we were quite impressed by Shannon's thought process, while feeling somewhat bothered at her juvenile gullibility.

In those first weeks following Shannon's release from the rehab center, Sue and I developed a morning ritual of getting up, taking the dog out, and going into Shannon's room for a quick chat. She was almost always awake, just lying in bed with her thoughts, while waiting for us to arise. Haley would jump on the bed and greet Shannon and we would ask her about her night.

We learned that Shannon was at her best in the morning. Her brain was refreshed, and she was typically very calm. By the end of each day, she was physically and mentally exhausted, and often became irritable and hard to please. Accordingly, we tried to conduct most of her learning activities in the morning, and dedicate the afternoons to simpler tasks, exercise, and rest. It was a pattern that worked well for us.

Samy left and Brian returned on Christmas Eve. As was our family ritual, Sue, Brian, Shannon, Kelley and I had a spaghetti dinner and read from the Bible. Then we decided to take a drive around Murfreesboro to look at the Christmas lights. The combination of motion and lights made Shannon nauseated and caused her to develop a major headache. It was another case of too much stimulation, and Shannon paid a heavy price. It took several hours to get rid of her headache and get settled for the night. We went to bed anxious about the headache, but fortunately she was fine on Christmas morning.

The last few days of December were very instructive. Shannon was exercising vigorously, and we discovered that the more she worked out, the better her outlook and mental acuity. Of course, all this exercise also caused her to experience pain in her shoulder, hip and foot, and raised her frustration level. We were constantly trying to find the correct balance of exercise and rest, and encouraged Shannon to walk instead of doing aerobics. It turned out to be a good compromise.

First, Shannon paced back and forth in the garage. When it was warmer, she would walk up and down the driveway. Later, when she was stronger, I walked with her around the neighborhood.

Just before New Year's, we had our weekly visits to Dr. Bradburn, Dr. Lowery and Dr. Hollis, all of which turned out well. Shannon liked all three and cooperated with them without hesitation. Each of them gave us good news. Dr. Lowery told us that he thought Shannon's collarbone would heal without surgery. Dr. Hollis told us that her jaw was mending nicely, and felt that he could remove the arch bars from her mouth in a few more days. Dr. Bradburn informed us that Shannon showed every indication that she would eventually regain 'normal range' brain function.

In spite of Dr. Bradburn's rosy prediction, it didn't take long for us to understand that *eventually* did not mean *now*. One evening, Brian, Shannon, Sue and I were sitting on the couch watching television, and I accidentally came across a program about brain injuries on the Discovery Channel. We watched intently as the narrator carefully explained how the neurons fired, how information is transmitted, how each segment of the brain fit with the others... and a thousand other bits of interesting information.

As I meticulously pointed out certain highlights to Shannon so that she could better understand what had happened to her, she would nod, acknowledge the data, and generally agree with my analysis.

"Dad, she doesn't have a clue what you're saying. She's completely faking it," admonished Brian.

"Maybe she's not getting it all, but it's a worthwhile effort," I replied.

"I'll bet she can't repeat back a single thing you told her. Go ahead, ask her a question."

Sadly, Brian was absolutely correct. Shannon didn't even know what day it was, much less have the capacity to assimilate technical information about brain function. It was a stark reality that tempered our optimism. In time, it was likely that Shannon would be able to comprehend new information, but for the present, it was a false hope. Before that sentinel moment, if we hadn't clearly understood that brain injury recovery takes a long time, we certainly did now.

❖❖❖

The first weeks of 1996 saw significant changes in Shannon's physical health and mental awareness. There was less pain in her collarbone, and the arch bars were removed from her teeth. Getting rid of the arch bars was a great relief... *after* it was over.

Shannon had been terrified by the thought of Dr. Hollis putting 'pliers' in her mouth and yanking out the braces that were imbedded in her gums. She feared both the pain and the potential for a bloodbath, not to mention the apprehension that her bottom jaw might fall off.

In spite of her trepidation, she sat calmly while Dr. Hollis worked. As it turned out, she need not have fretted so much. It took less than five minutes for him to complete the job... with no pain and no blood. And to Shannon's amazement, her jaw remained intact!

While Shannon was doing well overall, there were some trouble spots. She was still severely underweight, her collarbone still hurt, and she now had nerve pain radiating from her hip to her left foot.

We worked on her weight by adding a nutrition supplement to her milk... still *skim milk* I might add, and by giving her frequent snacks. It was a tedious process, however, because the more we fed her, the more she would exercise to get rid of the weight. It took many months before she regained her normal size.

The hip-to-foot pain was of some concern to us. We knew the nerves in her hip and/or back had been damaged, but we didn't know how long the pain would persist. It was disconcerting for Shannon because it bothered her when she sat in certain positions and when she tried to sleep.

Her 'salsa foot', as she referred to it, became a major source of complaint for the next two or three months. She would often roam the house at night, or soak her foot in a tub of cold water to relieve her discomfort. As it began to subside, we did have a lot of fun joking about it, though.

Some of these 'salsa foot' episodes are now pretty good 'war stories'.

By the middle of January, Shannon had been cleared for normal activity by all of her physicians. And with the exception of periodic visits to Dr. Bradburn, she was no longer doctor dependent. This lifted her spirits considerably.

Sue and Shannon established a routine of daily mental stimulation, designed to improve her memory, reasoning ability, and speech. They looked at Shannon's scrapbook for hours on end, talking about the people, places and events that marked her childhood, adolescence, teen and college years. They laughed about many of the normal behavioral issues confronted by parents and children, and they hugged a great deal. This was very effective therapy.

It was during one of these sessions that Shannon really cried for the first time since her accident. She was beginning to realize that she had moved to a new stage of life, and to her, the uncertain future was too painful to contemplate.

A second strategy for improving Shannon's comprehension and reasoning was to engage her in some form of debate. I would typically introduce a topic that was controversial, and ask questions that forced Shannon to take a position. I, of course, would almost automatically take a contrary one... forcing an argument. These debates were often heated, but were very helpful to both Shannon and the family in understanding her ability to assimilate information and formulate counter arguments. It was a risky approach because we didn't know how she would handle being boxed into a corner by logic. In spite of the aggravation these sessions caused, we concluded that it was an effective technique for brain stimulation.

These sessions also produced what one trained therapist calls an '*ah ha*', or a major revelation. Early on after Shannon awakened from her coma and began to interact with others, we saw little emotion and a lot of inhibition. It worried us that Shannon might say or do anything, and we openly wondered if she still had a sense of right or wrong. It was still a distressing thought until one of our mini-debates over a television news story.

The particulars of the discussion have long been forgotten, but Shannon clearly expressed a point of view that crime was wrong, and that punishment was a consequence of breaking the law. We could now see that Shannon did, in fact, comprehend the difference between good and bad, right and wrong, appropriate and inappropriate. It was a colossal realization.

Reading was another form of therapy that we tried to employ. Unfortunately, Shannon had never been a prolific reader, and no matter how much we encouraged it, she never showed much interest.

As a result of the economic challenges that faced us after the accident, Kelley volunteered to move back home while she finished her last two years of college. This allowed us to sell the condominium we had purchased for her a year earlier. It also looked like another therapeutic opportunity.

The apartment needed some repairs and a paint job before we could put it on the market, so Sue decided to tackle the task with Shannon's help. Needless to say, this was right up Shannon's alley. In a two week period, they worked together to replace the bathroom floor, clean kitchen appliances, and paint several rooms. All went well until one morning when Shannon accidentally knocked over a full can of white paint on a light brown carpet. Shannon looked at Sue, who returned the startled stare.

"*Oops*," muttered Shannon. They both laughed without restraint. This was another very telling sign that

Shannon was making significant mental progress. She recognized that a mistake had been made... but didn't go into her now customary rage.

They both knew they had to work quickly to scoop up the major spill, and carefully blot the remnants. In less than an hour, no one would have known the difference. More importantly, Shannon had handled adversity much better than she had in the previous weeks. We were now positive that it was only a matter of time before our ordeal was over, and Shannon would be her old self again. *Wrong!*

January 29, 1996 began as a crisp and sunny day with lots of promise. Sue and Shannon were just beginning their morning ritual at 7:45 a.m. when the telephone rang.

"Hello."

"Good morning, this is Sergeant Smith of the Lawrenceville, Georgia Police Department. May I speak with Mrs. Lloyd?"

"This is she."

"First, tell me how your daughter is doing?"

"She's doing very well. We have a long way to go, but she's making good progress. Thanks for asking."

"I'm certainly glad to hear that. Mrs. Lloyd, I'm sorry to be the one to bring you bad news after everything your family has been through."

"What kind of news?"

"Our lab tests showed that Shannon had a blood alcohol level of .12, which is over the legal limit in the State of Georgia. She's being charged with driving under the influence, and will have to face a trial in a few months."

Sue was stunned. In the first couple of days after the accident, we asked virtually everyone who was with Shannon that day if she had been drinking. Without exception, they said she had perhaps two glasses of beer in the last six hours before she and Brice had left Athens. Obviously, things didn't add up.

"Did you test Brice's alcohol level?"

"No, we didn't. We're not interested in the passenger's blood alcohol, only the driver."

"Is Shannon going to be arrested?"

"No, Shannon is not going to be arrested. You'll get a citation by certified mail in the next day or two, and she will have to appear in the Municipal Court at the appropriate time."

Sue's memory of the remainder of the conversation is vague. The only thing she can remember is that Sergeant Smith was very polite and kind, and seemed as pained as she was.

When Sue broke the news to Shannon, the patient went into hysterics. She promised that she had not been drinking. There had to be a mistake. Unfortunately, *there was no mistake*. We had been thrown another curve ball... and we were going to have to deal with it.

---NINE---

The Restless Period

Monday, January 29, 1996, 12:20 p.m.

I noticed the damage as soon as I rounded the curve and prepared to pull into our driveway:

...how could I possibly have missed that when I left for work this morning?... why would somebody *do* that? ...

The decorative lamps on top of the brick columns at the entrance to our driveway had been bashed, and there was glass everywhere. My anger got the best of me as I stormed into the hallway on my way to the kitchen to yell at somebody. Sue happened to be the victim of my tirade.

"Did you see what happened to the lights outside?"

That's as far as I got.

"I don't care about the lights right now. I got a call from the police in Lawrenceville this morning, and Shannon is being charged with DUI."

I was even more shocked at the news than she had been. I sat in disbelief as she carefully related her discussion with Sergeant Smith.

"Daddy, I didn't do it!" Shannon pleaded. "I didn't drink... I promise! They made a mistake... *they made a mistake*! She was so distressed that I dared not confront her. She actually *believed* she was innocent, even when the facts said otherwise. Our hopeful period was over. We had new issues to deal with... like a court case, hidden deficits, and an indeterminate future.

The urgency we felt over Shannon's recovery was no longer as intense as it had been when we first brought her home from the rehab center. It isn't that we cared less or had become complacent, but rather because we realized that Shannon's recovery was going to be more like a marathon than a sprint. We had to learn to pace ourselves to avoid emotional burnout. This meant trying to live as normal a life as possible.

The previous month had given us so many dramatic improvements that we had, at times, fallen into the trap of false euphoria, causing us to ignore many of the underlying disorders that still had to be confronted. The next few months brought us back to reality. While Shannon could function in a way that appeared to be normal to others, we knew the truth; *she was still an emotional and behavioral cripple.*

The major injury to Shannon's brain was in the left frontal lobe. We knew that this portion of the brain controls the speech process, but were now learning that it also affects the individual's perception, concentration and decision-making ability. All of which were noticeably impaired.

As the next few months passed, we gained a clearer picture of the deficits that needed attention. Perhaps the most visible was her emotional lability, or sudden, unexplained mood swings. One minute Shannon would be content and agreeable, and without any obvious change in her environment, she became irritable and argumentative. Since we didn't know what precipitated these mood swings, we couldn't prevent them, and for a few months it was like living with a volcano. We knew she was going to erupt, but we didn't know when, and we didn't know how much damage was going to occur when it bubbled over. The remedy for these episodes was physical exercise, either a workout or long walk.

The second most prevalent problem we faced was Shannon's inability to concentrate. Her attention span was limited, and she was easily distracted. We were able to make progress in this area relatively quickly, however, by giving her tasks that interested her. We put her drafting table upstairs where it was isolated and quiet, and encouraged her to draw. And draw she did.

In the next couple of months, Shannon re-accomplished many of the projects she had done in her graduate program in Interior Design, and also created new sketches from pictures in her architecture magazines. This led to marked improvement in all areas of concentration.

Another recognizable problem was a malfunction in Shannon's thought processes loosely called 'stereotypy of response'. That is, because of the frontal lobe injury, she could not quickly reply with independent thought during conversations. Accordingly, she used the same words or phrases repeatedly because they were easy to retrieve. This became very annoying, but there was simply no remedy except time. Sue and I often thought that if we heard the phrase 'call or contact' another time we would scream. Predictably, the problem got better as the weeks went by.

The most frustrating problem we faced was Shannon's bouts of restlessness, which lasted for almost three years. In retrospect, it's much easier to understand, but it was very difficult to deal with on a daily basis because we had no immediate cure. The remedy proved to be a combination of time, constructive engagement with the outside world, and a purpose for living.

Shannon, like her mother, had always been a planner and organizer, and disorder or vagueness would precipitate unbridled frustration. She was also action oriented. *Make a plan... and execute it.* That's how simple life was to her. Now, life had become too ambiguous and sedate. Shannon didn't know if she had enough memory or concentration to hold a job, so she couldn't plan. No plan meant no action... and for many months it was a vicious cycle of aimlessness, exasperation and restlessness.

Once we understood what was happening, we tried to establish short-term goals that we hoped would carry her to the ultimate goal of freedom, independence and normal function. We felt that if Shannon had some specific objectives to work toward, it would keep her mind off life's uncertainties.

We started with the computer, and a budding new technological invention called the Internet. It was a marvel because it functioned as an instant library and communications link to the outside world. Getting Shannon reconnected with her friends was just the tonic she needed to sharpen her mental skills and fight her edginess. Playing computer games also aided in improving her mental agility.

Daily e-mails with many of Shannon's high school and college friends were a blessing. This interaction made her feel that she was part of the outside world again and wasn't completely forgotten. She enjoyed the gossip and delighted in relating stories to us each day. However, there was also a price to be paid.

After a couple of months of following the progress of other people's lives, Shannon became discouraged because everyone else was going somewhere, while she was a 'shut in' with very limited potential. We had many conversations with her about patience during this period. All to no avail. She still felt like she was serving a life sentence.

As February began, we felt that it was time to find out if Shannon could cope with being home alone for short periods without supervision. Sue and I were scheduled to go to Minneapolis, Minnesota for a Medical Group Management Association (MGMA) conference planning meeting during the first week of February, and decided to let her stay at home during the day by herself. Haley, of course, would be her constant companion.

We were gone for four days. On Thursday and Friday, some of my co-workers visited during the day to be sure that Shannon was okay, while Kelley was home with her at night. On Saturday, Kelley took Shannon to the Mall for a while. We called often and worried a great deal. The mission proved to be a success. Shannon was pleased because we trusted her, and we were relieved that she had coped without incident.

The next target was a trip to Washington, D.C. in March. As President of MGMA, I was to deliver the opening address at the MGMA/AMA Leadership Conference on March 11th. Shannon helped me with my research, and she and Sue accompanied me to the session attended by several thousand physicians, medical administrators and government officials. Somewhere early in the presentation, I deviated from the script and began talking about the plight of the uninsured, and brought Shannon up on the stage while I told her story to the spellbound audience.

When I asked Shannon to come up on the dais, I really didn't know how she would react. She handled the pressure very well, and made her way down the isle and up to the platform without assistance. I had to admit, as I watched her walk toward me, that she was a tragic sight. Pale and thin, closely cropped hair, a bewildered look in her eyes, and an unsteady gait. Still, I was grateful that she was alive, and was alert enough to follow directions.

After the presentation, and throughout the conference, many physicians stopped me to ask questions and give me their assessment of her progress toward recovery. While each one saw something slightly different, they were all surprised that she could function at all. This was very heartening.

While I was in meetings, Sue and Shannon went to several of the museums and galleries of the Smithsonian Institution, and visited some other popular tourist destinations. Even though it was very cold and crowded, Shannon enjoyed the excursions immensely, and her attitude reflected her satisfaction. She was just happy to be on 'parole'. The trip proved to be an excellent reinforcement for her fragile psyche.

Three weeks later, Kelley and Shannon took an overnight trip to Birmingham for the wedding of one of Shannon's best high school friends. When they returned on Sunday, Kelley gave us a blow-by-blow account of the weekend activities. Shannon had enjoyed seeing many of her former classmates, but was clearly not her old self. She had been conversational, but had not been in the middle of the action like she used to be.

It was also the first time Shannon displayed another problem that was to plague her for three or four years... a lack of self-confidence. Prior to the accident, she enjoyed being the center of attention, and would tackle any social situation with gusto. Now she was unsure and reticent, and simply didn't have confidence in her ability to interact. It was, as Kelley described it, 'a bitter-sweet experience'. Still, it was another necessary step in the mending process.

It was during this period that I began to talk with Shannon about driving. For over a month, she steadfastly insisted that she would never drive a car again. The thought of having that responsibility was worrisome to her, but after trips to Washington and Birmingham, I felt that she was ready to get behind the wheel again. It was a Sunday morning at the end of March when I decided to push the issue.

"Shannon, I want you to go for a ride with me."

"Where are we going?"

"Nowhere in particular. Just a short drive around the block."

"Okay."

I don't think it occurred to her what I had in mind until we got to her car and I handed her the keys. She just stood there for a minute as if contemplating what she should do.

"Daddy, I don't want to drive."

"You're going to have to drive if you're ever going to be independent again. You might as well start now. "

"But, Daddy... I..."

"You want to be able to live on your own again, don't you?"

"Yes."

"Well, lets do it then."

"Okay."

Frankly, based on past conversations, I didn't think it would be that easy. Nonetheless, we got in the car and were on our way.

I don't know how nervous she was, but I was a basket case. She wobbled and weaved down the driveway and onto Irby Lane. While we never got over twenty-five miles an hour, and were never in any real danger, Shannon had difficulty maneuvering the car and staying on the right side of the road. The short trip of no more than a mile seemed like it took half an hour, and we were both relieved when it was over.

We repeated the process several times during the next month, gradually taking longer trips, including drives to and from the Clinic five miles away. Eventually we cleared that hurdle, and by May, Shannon was able to drive by herself again. Admittedly, we worried anytime she was gone, but we really had little choice. Returning her to adulthood meant that she had to have the freedom of movement.

The budding trees and blooming flowers of spring were accompanied by an emerging new Shannon. She became preoccupied with the lost days and months since the accident, and she incessantly talked about the need to find out where she had been, who she really was now, and what the future would hold.

We spent many hours talking with Shannon about details of her graduation from the Savannah College of Art & Design in late May, her move to Marietta, Georgia, her job at the furniture company, her friends, and the events that occurred the day before the accident.

She was absolutely obsessed with the time between November 12, 1995 and late February of 1996, and wanted to know everything. Most pointedly, she wanted to know exactly why she was driving Brice's car, and precisely what happened to cause the accident. Unfortunately, we couldn't give her any satisfactory answers.

She was so disturbed about her lack of recall that we took her back to Dr. Bradburn in early April for a six-month evaluation. He answered her questions and carefully explained some of the simple mechanics of brain function so she could understand the nature of the healing activity taking place within her head. He also tried to reassure her that she had progressed very well.

Dennis Bradburn's communication style was always direct and to the point... and he never minced words or talked down to patients. His last comments to Shannon at the end of the visit reflected that approach, and are indelibly etched in my memory to this day.

"Shannon, you suffered a severe head injury, from which you've made a remarkable recovery. You are now functioning in the *normal range*, and there's no reason why you can't work, have a social life, get married, and have children some day. You aren't the same person you were before the accident, but that doesn't mean you're a lesser person. You're just different than you were before. Pretty soon you'll be the person you are now... *or* the one you're going to be. Most of the healing is now complete."

To us, that was a sobering reality. Yes, Shannon could perform assigned tasks, could remember facts and figures and carry on reasonable conversations, but her perceptions of the world, her impatience, and her seeming immaturity were alarming. Shannon left Dr. Bradburn's office full of expectation, while Sue and I were palpably less optimistic. Our plans were unaltered though. We would just continue the process of rehabilitation. After all, what else could we do?

While our primary focus in the first few months of 1996 was on Shannon's rehabilitation, by necessity we also devoted a substantial amount of time to the legal issues surrounding the accident. Shortly after being notified of the DUI charges, I called a fraternity brother who practiced law in Atlanta. He referred us to a colleague who specialized in this particular area of the law.

Janice Schrader was a good choice. She was always positive, she kept us informed during every step of the process, and offered helpful and appropriate advice during the entire legal proceedings. There were some difficult moments, however, because of the potential penalties of a guilty verdict.

Several times during March and April, Shannon became completely hysterical over the prospect of going to jail. Her ranting and raving always ended with, "I'll kill myself before I'll go to jail!" We continually tried to tell her not to jump to conclusions; but it was futile. She worried constantly about being sent to jail for life, in spite of our reassurances.

In early April, Janice Schrader called with good news. The Solicitor of the Municipal Court had suggested a 'nolo contendere' plea, which would result in a fine of seven hundred dollars, forty hours of community service, and the completion of a defensive driving course. She would also be on probation for two years. More importantly to Shannon, she would not have to appear in court.

Writing a check for the fine was straightforward, and arranging for her community service at Middle

Tennessee Medical Center was easy enough. Traffic school was another matter.

Getting Shannon into a Defensive Driving course in the Nashville area was extremely difficult because there were a limited number of State sanctioned programs available, and because all of them were solidly booked for the next several months. However, through Sue's persistence, we finally found a facility in Smyrna, Tennessee, about fifteen miles from Murfreesboro.

The course was held for three hours, once per week, for four weeks. We knew it was going to be difficult for Shannon the minute we drove up to the building for the first session. The gravel parking lot was full of old jalopies with dented fenders, broken windows, bald tires, and obscene or racially insensitive bumper stickers. The mostly male owners milling around outside the building were perfect matches for their vehicles. Shannon was to learn that almost every one of them were chronic offenders… and didn't even have valid driver's licenses!

Needless to say, Shannon was both offended and humiliated by having to associate with these 'criminals' on a weekly basis. The course was a complete farce. During one class, a guy sitting next to Shannon actually asked her if she wanted to skip out at the break and go down the street to a bar. In any event, we were relieved when it was over and she received her certificate of completion.

One of my life philosophies is that no experience is wasted… *it can always be used as a bad example.* This was certainly one of those times. This experience taught Shannon that she didn't want to end up like so many of her wayward classmates.

It would take until the middle of June for Shannon to fulfill all the requirements set forth by the Municipal Court in Lawrenceville, Georgia, and for the case to be closed. Finally, the black legal cloud that had covered us for almost six months was over.

By all accounts, Shannon had made an amazing and miraculous recovery. She wasn't perfect, but she was functional and still progressing. She now wanted to go back to the Gwinnett Medical Center, meet the people who had saved her life, and see the ICU and Room 616. This would help her to close the memory gap that troubled her so much. We agreed that it was a good idea.

Sue, Shannon and I met Samy in Atlanta on a cool and rainy Friday and made our way over to the hospital. It was an eerie experience. The three of us took turns showing Shannon everything from the emergency room to the cafeteria. We told her many stories about people and events during the time that she lay comatose in the ICU or immobile in her hospital room. It was as if we were tour guides at Disney World, talking about all of the interesting rides and sights. Shannon listened intently, but dispassionately.

When we arrived at the ICU and the Nursing Station on the sixth floor, there were hugs and excited conversation. Everyone recognized Sue, Samy and me... but didn't have a clue who Shannon was because she looked so much different. Believe it or not, the introductions were awkward. Shannon didn't know how to react. She politely thanked them for saving her life and taking care of her, but she was unable to summon up the emotions the rest of us felt.

Overall, the reunion was a success, if for no other reason than it gave Shannon some visual background for so many of the events we had talked about. It was another key element in closing the memory gap.

Shannon's major goal during the first half of 1996 was to regain enough strength and mental acuity to be part of Jennifer Beaulieu (Behrens') wedding party in the spring. Prior to the accident, Shannon had been helping Jenn with the planning, and the thought of not being able to participate in her best friend's wedding was devastating. She was, therefore, determined to do whatever was necessary to be in Birmingham, Alabama on May 4th. Goals are powerful motivators, and we used this one many times when Shannon seemed to lose her focus.

Shannon thought she was now ready for her coming out party, and vowed not to sit in the background as she had at her friend Tracey's wedding in March. She was true to her word. She talked, she danced, and she joked with her friends. The problem was that her communication deficits were highly magnified, and at times she was truly a pathetic figure.

Jennifer and Paul were extremely gracious and understanding, as were most of her old friends, but Sue, Kelley and I were, at times very uncomfortable. Shannon, on the other hand, had a ball!

More than a year after the accident, Shannon wrote the following in her journal. It shows remarkable insight about that weekend.

...I missed out on all of Jennifer's wedding showers. I had helped her and worked with her on wedding plans before the accident. I missed out on all the fun. I was still in the wedding as co-maid of honor with Stephanie. The bridesmaid luncheon was fun. The wedding was fun. Now that I look at the pictures, I looked sick, but I wouldn't have missed that day...

---TEN---

The Identity Crisis

Thursday, June 13, 1996, 9:45 a.m.

The big day was here. Shannon was going back to work. As Sue dropped her off at Hickory Hollow Mall in Nashville, Shannon was having her doubts:

...I really have mixed feelings... I'm so nervous... I haven't been to work in almost eight months... can I do this? ... what do I look like? ... what do they expect from me? ... do I need this? ... *do I really need this*? ...

The answer was yes. I needed to get out of the house because I was doing nothing challenging. I spent time drawing, exercising, walking, doing yard work, going grocery shopping, and worrying about my future.

In my mind, I knew I could do retail work, even though that's not what I wanted to do forever. I did it before, during graduate school and after initially moving to Atlanta. A few years earlier, after only a month I had been promoted to Manager. It was easy... if I remember correctly.

The furniture store in Marietta, Georgia had recommended me to the Hickory Hollow Mall branch, so I decided to give it a try. I thought working in the same environment would help me regain some memory and confidence. In fact, it did. In the following two months, I really enjoyed working with the customers, and I was very successful at selling merchandise. On the other hand, I spent much of my time frustrated because of the way the store was run.

That first day, my manager, Rachel, gave me a brief rundown of supplies, inventory and other employees. I forgot much of what she said five minutes after she told me. That particular day, only three employees were scheduled to work, and I admit I was a little scared.

137

...will it be the same as it had been? ... will I know the right answers to customer questions? ...

I quickly found the answer to those questions. I saw a customer looking at accessories so I walked over and asked her if I could help her locate something. She said no and basically walked away. I was a little hurt.

...did I say something wrong?... is it the way I look?...

Soon after that, another couple asked my opinion and wanted to know about a particular piece. What was its purpose? Style? Cost? Availability? Other pieces it works with? I jumped on that. Technically it was a basic side table, but I created a casual working environment for the customer's home office. Somehow the creative/design side of my mind came into play without much forced stimulation. He eventually purchased the side table, a lamp, a few prints, small accessories and a desk and chair set. After completing that transaction, I knew I would be fine.

Sue and I were apprehensive about how Shannon would react under the stress of fast paced interaction with customers and having to take orders from a supervisor. We feared that her inability to consistently phrase sentences correctly, her impatience, and her volatility might be a turn-off to customers and management. If Shannon's communication deficits bothered customers, it didn't show in her sales results. Once again, she was a top sales associate... just as she had been before. We never saw any evidence of conflict with her manager either.

We worried constantly, however, because we never knew when the volcano would erupt. Apparently, Shannon was perceptive enough to avoid clashes at work, and waited until she got home to complain and argue. We had plenty of squabbles! I found that the best way to calm her was to let her harangue for as long as she liked. I engaged in arguing as little as I could, and I didn't try to calm her. She did that by herself. It was actually pretty simple if I displayed some patience. After awhile she just got tired and gave up.

I worked daily at the Hickory Hollow branch during June and July. After only working one month, I knew I wanted to be back in Atlanta. *I had to be.* I wouldn't feel like me or complete until I was where I was appreciated, had friends, and really enjoyed my co-workers.

Working in Tennessee wasn't that much fun. Most of my co-workers were there for an income. I was there because I knew the merchandise and thought I was helping customers. During those two months, I also worked at another Nashville branch store. My manager told me I knew exactly what to do and the right way to do it, so I was asked to help. Honestly, I did things the way I thought they needed to be done. I never had any handbook or instructions. It was what I remembered being taught as I grew up.

It didn't take very long for us to settle into a new routine. Shannon worked four or five days a week for six hours or less, would come home and exercise, eat dinner, and go to bed at 8:30 p.m. or so. The sustained mental activity required at work exhausted her, and once in bed, she slept for ten to twelve hours. We had learned from raising a hearing impaired child that concentration causes mental fatigue, and sleep is a very good remedy.

It was on Shannon's days off that she constantly whined and complained about her life, became irritable, and showed a great deal of immaturity. We noticed when Shannon first began regaining her faculties that many of her behaviors were very juvenile. Her physicians and therapists assured us that this was a normal phase in brain injury recovery, and that over time she should re-mature.

They were right to a point, but it seemed to us that she had reached a plateau as a fourteen year old. She functioned well enough on routine matters, but if things didn't go exactly her way, she would pout and complain. The task of having to contend with a perpetual teenager was very trying.

On the first couple of weekends after Shannon returned to work, Sue and I drove the thirty miles to Hickory Hollow Mall and spent time browsing in the various stores. In reality, we were there to see first hand how Shannon was doing in her communication with customers. Having known her before the accident, it was easy to spot differences in her abilities, but to the casual observer, she seemed perfectly normal. This helped lessen our worry... that is, until Shannon was assigned to do inventory from late afternoon until midnight at the end of June.

"Mom, I have to do inventory from 4:00 p.m. to midnight on Sunday, Monday and Tuesday," Shannon announced at breakfast on Saturday morning.

"Shannon, do you really have to do that? Can't they get someone else? We're not particularly in favor of you being out so late at night, or driving home alone at that hour."

"It's part of my job Mom, and I know more about it than any of my co-workers do, anyway. I'll be okay."

Then I chimed in. "We'll agree to let you do that under one condition. You need to call us before you leave the Mall each night."

"I'll be okay. Don't worry so much."

Sunday and Monday nights went fine. She completed her work around midnight, called to let us know she was on her way, and was home in forty-five minutes. Tuesday night was another matter.

We went to bed around 10:30 p.m. and I fell asleep quickly. I woke up at 12:45 a.m. and realized that Shannon had not called. Sue and I briefly discussed what we should do, and I decided to call the store. No answer. I redialed the number. No answer. Now we were about to panic.

"I'm going up to Hickory Hollow and see if I can find her," I said to Sue as I put on a shirt and shorts.

"Be careful."

At approximately 1:00 a.m. I was out the door. I decided that I would retrace her normal route, and would watch the other side of the highway as I drove so I wouldn't miss her if she were already on her way home.

I tried to convince myself that I was being overly anxious and that she was probably tied up in the warehouse and couldn't hear the telephone. I saw no accidents on the way to the Mall, but couldn't help worrying about the possibility that someone had abducted her as she left.

...why didn't she call? ... no call means she's still there... okay, it's fine... things just ran late, that's all...

As much as I tried, I couldn't control my heart rate. I arrived at the Mall at 1:35 a.m. and drove around the entire parking lot. My heart sank. There were very few cars... and Shannon's wasn't among them.

I located a security guard and told him I was looking for my daughter. I related our story to him and he became equally concerned. He graciously opened the door to the back of the store and it was completely dark. At that point, I simply didn't know what to do except return home, hoping that she would somehow be there.

As I pulled into the driveway at 2:45 a.m., I spotted Shannon's car parked by the garage, and saw lights on in the kitchen. I was furious and relieved at the same time. I walked in the door and Shannon quickly apologized. She had forgotten to call us until she was out the door, and couldn't get back inside once the door closed behind her. The next day, we got her a cell phone.

During this whole episode, with a new job and actually driving a car again, I still questioned who I was. I didn't know if I worked so proficiently because it was as basic as knowing the back of my hand, or if I did it just to try to impress people.

I was full of strange feelings. The best way to explain it is by comparing myself to a defendant's thoughts in a well-known television series, *Law & Order*. I had feelings of unwanted guilt, constant surveillance, and being forever known for my last move... a mistake in judgment. I was completely paranoid.

...did I do it? ... was I there? ... how did they find out about that? ... who saw me? ...

Many days I would talk to myself in the mirror:

"...how do you feel today? ... do you look better today? ...how old are you today? ...what will you complain about today? ... can I do it? ... why does it work that way, and how am I supposed to make it work? ..."

It was a time that I expected all these burning questions to be answered. Sometimes I thought that I could answer myself fully and correctly. At other times, I wasn't so sure. I felt that *if* I could only answer these questions, then everything would eventually be okay.

I wondered if I was smart. I wondered if I was fun to talk to or be around. I wondered if the way I acted or what I said was respectable or proper. At age twenty-four and a half, I knew I wasn't really acting or doing what everyone else my age did. I was at my parents' home, not my own. I never went anywhere except the grocery store. I didn't have any friends in Murfreesboro to call.

I knew I had a Masters' Degree in Interior Design, but I also had puzzling questions:

...how did I get that? ... why? ... I wasn't doing anything related to what I studied...

All the while I just felt like I was going in circles. Between doctor visits, procedures, and the ongoing court case, I couldn't find equilibrium. I was meeting strange people, I was dependent, and I had no social life. I didn't cope very well, and I wondered if I ever would.

Nothing I did was as good as I think it should have been. I kept hearing Mom and Dad discuss how I talked or reacted. They didn't know I heard them. I was a little sneaky... much like a fourteen year old. I didn't use the correct words to tell a story or make a complaint. I copied many things I said either within the last hour or past two days. I was okay... *but could I function out in the world without them there?*

I was very confused at what was happening to me. Everyone told me what had happened many times over. I didn't believe it most of the time. I even had good 'comebacks':

"I forgot that. When was that? I missed out on that. You never told me that. I threw that away. It must be in a box in the attic or in Atlanta. I'm fine. The storyline you guys are using would make a pretty good movie. How about a Broadway Show? I'll audition for the part. "

It was all a charade. I was completely unsure of myself and scared to death.

It was a constant struggle at that time just to overcome my own fears and emotions. I wasn't able to accept anything that actually happened to me. *And I didn't want anyone to know.*

While Shannon was trying to find herself, I tried to carry on as normally as I could. It was July, and I had places to go and obligations to fulfill. Actually, the diversion was good therapy for me. In addition to my daily responsibilities of running a medical clinic, I was at the peak of my duties as President of MGMA.

I traveled to and from our Headquarters in Englewood, Colorado a couple of times; and Sue and I attended regional conferences in Asheville, North Carolina; Traverse City, Michigan; and Nashville. We also spent a week in Minneapolis attending the Association's Board of Directors meeting. This, of course, left Shannon at home with Kelley and Haley for most of the month.

We checked in frequently during our travels to be sure that everything was on an even keel. Fortunately, there were no major problems, and life seemed relatively normal. Throughout July, Shannon began insisting that she needed to go back to Atlanta and resume her life. I had reservations... Sue was adamantly opposed!

A sample of our many discussions on the issue went like this:

"Pretty soon it will be time for us to let Shannon move back to Atlanta where she has a familiar job and friends," I suggested.

"She's not ready, " replied Sue.

"When do you think she will be ready? "

"Not for several more months... *if ever*. First, I don't think she can cope with the combination of traffic, the mobs of people, maintaining an apartment, and the responsibility of a full time job. "

"We can't keep her here forever. She's done pretty well at the furniture store and has taken care of the house while we've been gone. I think we need to give her a chance to live independently again. "

"She's not ready. Besides, how are we going to pay for her living expenses? We're already paying her school loans, car payment, insurance premiums and medical bills *now*. How will we *ever* be able to take on apartment rent, utilities and other expenses? Her salary won't cover a third of them. "

"We'll manage somehow. If we don't let her go, she'll be dependent on us for the rest of her life. Besides, she'll make our lives miserable if we don't give her a chance. "

"I just don't think she's capable of handling the daily responsibilities of living... cooking, doing laundry, paying bills, and dealing with all the commotion in the Atlanta rat race."

"I know she's not as mentally agile as she needs to be, but if we don't give her a chance, it won't ever get better. "

This debate went on for more than a month. Sometimes, when Shannon was included in the conversations, she became very agitated and insistent. Her constant refrain was:

"I can't get my life back until I move 'home'."

It was hard to argue that point. After all, she was almost twenty-five years old, and was functioning as well as most other adults in society... at least according to her physician. Her perceptions might have been somewhat askew, and her communication skills may not have been very polished at times, but wasn't that pretty representative of most of us, too?

Eventually, Sue gave in because '*everybody beat me to death*'. She realized that we couldn't shield Shannon from the world around her indefinitely, but like all concerned mothers, she wanted to try.

After my constant whining and begging to Mom and Dad, I was finally told I would be allowed to move back 'home'. I researched apartments and housing in Atlanta as soon as I had the opportunity. Having that much incentive and drive, I found the perfect apartment, packed all my belongings, called old contacts, and was more than welcomed back to my old store. I moved back to Atlanta on August 16, 1996.

I would be on my own again... back in *my* environment, back to *my* old life, having fun, going places, being somebody! Why shouldn't I? After all... *there was nothing wrong with me anyway!* Or so I thought.

---ELEVEN---

The Great Escape

Friday, August 16, 1996, 1:15 p.m.
  ... free at last... free at last...

Knowing Shannon, that's exactly how she felt when we arrived at the Summit Village apartments in Marietta, Georgia after the three-hour drive from Murfreesboro.

  ... oh, no, what have I done? ...

That's definitely what I thought as it dawned on me that we would be leaving Shannon here alone in a just forty-eight short hours.

At Shannon's insistence, we had risen early, packed my Jeep and her car with boxes, clothes and a few pieces of small furniture, and were on our way to her new home. While Sue rode with Shannon in her car, I was alone in the Jeep... and had plenty of time to question my judgment about letting Shannon move back to Atlanta. After fighting the traffic near her apartment complex, I was sure I had made the wrong decision. Once again, Sue was right. Shannon wasn't ready for this. Unfortunately, it was too late to turn back.

Shannon's new apartment was on the third floor overlooking a large lake; a one-bedroom flat with a nice drawing room off the living room. She had made a good selection. It was in a less congested area of the complex, and was quiet and secure.

After unloading both vehicles, we had some lunch and went looking for a bed and some other furniture. It was then that I produced twenty-one hundred-dollar bills and turned them over to Shannon. The money was a gift from the physicians and staff of the Murfreesboro Medical Clinic. They collected it while she was still lying unconscious in the Gwinnett Medical Center nine months before. Shannon was genuinely touched.

"Why would they do that for someone they barely know, Daddy?" she asked with tears in her eyes.

"Because they care," was all I could muster. "Simply because they care."

During that afternoon we managed to buy a bed and frame, a dining room table and matching chairs, a lamp table, and a coffee table. Shannon was very animated and engaged in the process. So much so, in fact, that her words ran together and I had to constantly tell her to slow down and think before trying to speak.

The next morning we went to another couple of stores and found a very nice oversized sofa for her living room. I was rather amazed after we finished our shopping spree that we had furnished her apartment with some quality pieces for around $2,500. It didn't hurt that everything we purchased had either been on sale or had been bought from her own furniture store, where she received a significant discount. Shannon, like her mother, was still the consummate bargain hunter.

We chose this particular weekend for the move because it coincided with a fraternity reunion in the Atlanta area. Since my brother, Ken, was also a member of the same fraternity, he flew in from Houston for the event. He met us at the apartment on Saturday afternoon and was astonished at the progress Shannon had made since he had last seen her just before Christmas. We were pleased and relieved that an impartial observer thought she looked and acted 'normal'.

Sue and Shannon stayed at the apartment on Saturday evening while Ken and I were attending the function. It was a stormy night. Not because of the weather, but because Shannon wanted to assemble the entertainment center for the TV and VCR by herself... and wanted to arrange furniture and accessories without her mother's perceived interference. They eventually reached an accommodation and the clash ended without major cmotional damage. It was this kind of behavior that worried us the most.

The weekend went by very quickly, and all too soon, it was time for Sue and I to leave for Tennessee. As we said our goodbyes and got in the Jeep, Shannon stood at the curb and waved at us with a wistful smile. It was reminiscent of another day almost exactly nineteen years prior. Before I realized it, I was laughing out loud through my tears.

"What is it?" Sue asked with a puzzled look on her face.

"Oh, nothing," I replied as I wiped away the tears. "I was just thinking about our Las Vegas vacation."

It took her a few seconds to make the connection, and then she joined me in the laughing fit.

In August of 1977 we lived in Redlands, California... a community of approximately thirty-five thousand people, just off Interstate 10 a little over half way between Los Angeles and Palm Springs. Brian was eight, Shannon was about to turn six, and Kelley was just short of two years old. Our house was one of four on a circle just off a semi-main street. Two of the other three families had children comparable to ours, and the third family had children old enough to baby-sit for the rest of us. It was a neat little package.

It was a Friday morning, and Sue and I were leaving for our first vacation in several years... a short weekend trip to Las Vegas. Sue had meticulously organized the trip and the baby-sitter, prepared and labeled all the meals, set out the kids' clothes for the next four days, and essentially made sure no detail was overlooked.

We were full of anxiety as we backed out of the driveway since we had never before left our children with anyone except their grandparents. We were also a little melancholy, and somewhat concerned that the kids would be frightened at our leaving. Brian was already busy with a friend, and never gave us a second thought. Predictably, Kelley was crying... a pattern that still exists today.

Shannon, of course, commanded the spotlight. As we drove away, we looked back to see her jump up, click her heels together perfectly, and whoop, "*Yippee... Yippee... Yippee!*"

That day, we laughed through our tears half way to Las Vegas. Today, we relived that moment... although for a much different reason.

I was anxious for the day to get started, and I purposely got up early and made some noise so Mom and Dad would get up. Before we left I wrote the following in my journal:

...what a day I won't forget... my first day of 'freedom' since my accident... it resembles the first day I headed off to college and set up my new life away from home... I didn't sleep at all last night... too excited... by the end of the day, I'll have my own place... I can decorate, build, and clean as I wanted to, not as asked or expected... I can have my friends come over to eat, watch movies, plan more adventures, and catch up on the past nine months... I have high hopes... I have so much to do to 'get up to speed' with everything I haven't done or missed... I used to always be ahead of the pack, well prepared, ready to try something new... *I will be again*, just wait...

The weekend was busy with activity. *I loved it!* After each piece of furniture was delivered and set up, I felt more complete. I actually had a purpose again. I was back in the State I loved, closer to many friends, had my own living environment, and was closer to the career connections I needed to become the successful designer I had written about in my past journals and seen through the work in my portfolio.

By moving, I realized that no one would be there when I woke up or returned from work. That made me feel alone, but I was comforted by the memory that I had lived by myself in graduate school with no problems. I wanted to make a life again. I was tired of analyzing me. I would much rather be talking to my friends about their problems. I started thinking that my new home was my office. I could talk, create, draw, build, exercise, and do whatever I wanted to, whenever I wanted to.

On Sunday as Mom and Dad were leaving, I started to get a little teary-eyed. They had helped me. They listened when I needed to complain. And I did get a daily hug or two. They were family. But then again, I could do it by myself. I had to prove it.

...who cares anyway... I'm on my own again! ...

The next seventeen months were some of the most challenging of our collective lives. Sue and I constantly fretted about Shannon's welfare, and grieved for her disappointments and loneliness. The combination of too much stimulation, perceived failure, disillusionment with her friends, and just plain confusion, turned Shannon into the active volcano we feared. She spent much of her time in a full-scale eruption of emotions.

In spite of her unhappiness and fragile psyche, she did hold a job and carry out the essential activities of life. Accordingly, we couldn't pull the financial plug and force her to come back to Tennessee. It seemed to us that our only recourse was to let her remain in Atlanta and try to work her way through this difficult period. We gave her encouragement and emotional support, and let her know she was always welcome at home. But we openly questioned whether or not we were doing the right thing.

Shortly after her move, we were introduced to another common consequence of a brain injury. It is called 'flooding', and although we didn't recognize it as such before, we had seen it in small increments a number of times previously. Now it was a major problem.

This phenomenon occurs when the individual becomes so overwhelmed by options, alternatives or simple data that the brain loses its ability to process information. The result is that the problem-solving mechanism becomes severely impaired, and the individual is unable to make even the simplest decision. Multitasking is absolutely impossible. The individual may find him or herself standing in the kitchen unable to decide whether or not to go to the bedroom, bathroom or living room, or what to do when they get there.

As far as we know, Shannon's most severe episode of 'flooding' occurred while she was in her car... a potentially disastrous situation. Fortunately, she pulled over into a parking lot and called me because she was conditioned enough to believe I would know what to do. More about that later.

While there were some positive developments during this time, more often we lived from one emotional crisis to another. In spite of our efforts not to worry, we did not look forward to the telephone ringing. We knew if it was Shannon, we were more than likely in for another emotional roller coaster ride.

My first few months back in Atlanta were a time of soul searching and trying to rediscover myself. I had been out of touch for nine months, and I was very unsure of who I was and how I was supposed to act.

I worked at the furniture store; I arranged and decorated my apartment; I tried to reconnect with friends from school and work; and I worried about fitting-in again. The work and decorating went fine; renewing friendships and fitting-in were a problem. Regardless of how hard I tried, I just couldn't find a comfortable social life.

Notes from my journal in late August reveal just how bad things were:

...Here I am sitting in my own place. Why am I upset? Or the better question to ask myself, what genuine reasons do I have to be upset? I am totally a nut case. My feelings change like the weather... rain or shine, 50/50 every day. How am I supposed to live with that? Who would want to be with me? If I am just associating my feelings and thoughts with the accident, I need to know what effects it will have on my life now and in the future. I don't know who to talk to. I try to accept it all and put it in the past. I learned from it. Will that help me with my fast, wild decisions? I wish it never happened in the first place. I feel very lucky and am happy to be here, but my problem is what I constantly think about. The priority seems to be becoming who I was. Everyone liked me then. I was successful then. I liked myself then. I had friends then. I had plans for the future then. Dreams were coming true then. I have no self-confidence now. Mom and Dad tell me to talk to them anytime about anything. I don't want to tell them these things... I'm just another disappointment...

One positive aspect resulting from my tragedy was that Brian and I talked more. We lived in the same city, but it was hard to see each other very often, so we talked several times a week by telephone. We had deep conversations. Hour after hour passed, and we talked about everything imaginable. I know it was good for me; and I think it was good for Brian, too.

My plan was to continue working at the furniture store while I looked for a job in my chosen field of Interior Design. I was still a member of the IIDA (International Interior Design Association), and I thought the best place to start was to attend the monthly meetings and get involved. Most people seemed to remember me... at least my name. The meetings were informal, but there was one recurring theme that I really hated. *Do you have the right connections?* I didn't, and I resented it. Still, I tried to fit in.

I met with a few IIDA members. Each of them told me they were glad I was okay and would look to see if any openings appeared that I could do. Meeting with these associates felt like interviews daily. I was so nervous.

...what did I sound like? ... did I make sense? ... did I repeat myself? ...

Lucky enough, I was invited to the mid-year planning retreat at the beginning of 1997. I felt that it would be a sure fit to my design world. I was to be involved with twenty members of IIDA away from the business world, and thought that maybe it would entice my creative mind. In spite of my trying, it just never worked out.

I was glad to be back in Georgia for the beginning of the college football season. I loved it, and I felt better being involved. I was invited and didn't turn down the chance to watch college football with my old college buddies because it helped me forget my insecurities. It was also depressing, however, because I could see that they were all moving on in their lives... and I was not. Again, notes from my journal tell the story:

...How? Why? When? These are the same questions I ask myself every day. I am trying to find an answer to why I feel so lost. I am outside of everything. I used to be a part of everything. Now, I never am. I have no self-esteem. I think about what people think of me. I get tired of those questions because no one can answer all of them. What would life be like if these questions were answered? No surprises or life at all. Why is it that I answer some questions with more questions? I only make sense to me and even that doesn't make sense. I didn't plan or do much this month. No big days. Just work at the store and think about what I would like to be doing. I talk to myself, write in a journal, talk to my fish, and hope things will happen for me soon...

We visited Shannon a couple of times in the first few months after she moved back to Atlanta, and were particularly impressed at how well she had done in painting and decorating her apartment. She had truly turned a standard looking unit into *her* home, a place that reflected the personality we had always known. We now knew she was equipped physically and organizationally to manage a job and her own household.

We also saw the other side... high impatience, frustration, self-deprecation, and a completely unbalanced perception of the world around her. She kept asking the question, "Am I a real person?" There was nothing we could say or do to make her feel better. We wanted to believe that eventually some good things would happen to her to lift her spirits, but we fretted that she may never get any better, and that some day the frustrations would engulf her. Time would either be an ally or an enemy... we just didn't know which.

We were confident that Shannon could cope with a repetitive routine, but did she have the mental agility to deal with the unfamiliar and unpredictable? Her first test was a plane trip to Minneapolis for the Annual Conference of the Medical Group Management Association in mid October. I was concluding my presidency of the Association, and Shannon was going to have to attend many functions and deal with crowds of people anxious to see how she was doing.

"Shannon, everybody is going to want to talk to you. They will ask a million questions about how and what you're doing, what your plans are for the future, how you like Atlanta, and God knows what else. Don't get flustered. Stay calm, take a deep breath, and talk slowly. You don't have to entertain them. Just talk like you're talking to me. If you begin to 'flood', just excuse yourself and come back to the room for a little while and collect your thoughts."

"I'll be okay, Dad. I won't embarrass you."

155

Her answer said it all. She lacked confidence in her ability to communicate spontaneously, but she was determined to try. Shannon was received warmly, and my colleagues overlooked any communication difficulties. They were surprised that she was as fluent and agile as she was. My close friends who knew Shannon could see that she was more guarded and reticent, but for the most part, they felt she handled herself admirably. It was an important test, and showed that she could master a social situation... at least with her family present.

Before I knew it, the calendar read November 11th, 1996... three hundred and sixty four days after the accident. I realized that the next day would be the one-year anniversary of the event that changed my life, but I couldn't remember any details. I had a weird feeling because I just couldn't visualize what happened that day, or any of the events that had dominated the last year. I felt lost.

I wanted to talk to Mom and Dad and thank them for all they had done for me, but I couldn't bring myself to call them. I just didn't want them to relive that horrible experience. Late in the day, however, they called me. It was important for me to understand what had happened, and they were my only reliable source of information. While I will *never* fully understand what happened, I'm more comfortable today because I have almost five years of new memories, and no longer have the need to focus on that period of my life.

I was alone most of the time when I wasn't working. I would visit my grandmother on Sundays when I could, I attended a neighborhood church, I strolled around Marietta, went to some street festivals and arts & crafts shows, and I exercised a lot just to pass the time. I also continued to try to find a job in the design world... unsuccessfully.

...why can't I just live a normal life? ...

While my activities might have been normal for other people, it wasn't the old me. I liked action and activity, and I liked being involved with lots of people. Because I was no longer 'in circulation', I constantly analyzed and overanalyzed myself. As I look back, it's a miracle that I didn't go crazy.

The next few months were confused. I was frustrated because I had no career, few friends, and lots of worries. Again, my journal provides some insights into my thinking at the time:

January, 1997: **...I feel like I have no drive... no reachable goals... do I have intelligence? ... can I do what I did before? ... I am twenty-five, not fifteen---and act fifteen, not twenty-five...**

February, 1997: **...I don't know what I need except calm myself down... where is my self-calming, patient self... gone or hiding? ... am I expecting too much? ...**

March, 1997: **...The single solemn life is not terrible... sometimes lonely, but I have to accept it and deal with it... That is part of the plan of my life... accept it, continue and move on... have my hour of sorrow and get on with it... That is the plan... I'll make it work... it's all on me... I have to do it or I am nothing...**

In March, I made a decision to take action to change my life. I bought a new computer, I worked on improving my CAD (computer aided design) skills, I sent resumes to dozens of design firms, and vowed to improve my self-image. April was to be a breakthrough month.

I began a four-week refresher class in CAD at Chattahoochee Technical College in early April so I could demonstrate that I was qualified for a design job. I had a few interviews during the month, and was able to get a part-time job at Casablanca Design in Marietta. My plan was to continue working at the furniture store while I built up my hours in the new job. Eventually, I hoped to be full time at Casablanca.

In addition to my work activities, I participated in planning for my college roommate's wedding. Kim Sothen (Black) was the same as always... playful, happy, friendly and positive, and she didn't shy away from me the way some of my other friends seemed to do.

I also attended the spring graduation exercises of the Savannah College of Art & Design at the end of May. I was nervous about seeing some of my former professors and classmates who knew about the accident, but they all welcomed me with open arms. *Finally*, things were beginning to look better to me.

"Mr. Lloyd, I think it's Shannon on the telephone."

That wasn't unusual, because she often called me at work to talk about either the good or bad things that were happening in her life. It was just part of the process. This call was different, however.

"Hi honey. Are you alright?"

I was greeted with hysterical sobbing, and it was almost two minutes before she could utter a coherent word.

"Daddy, I got fired by Casablanca..."

My heart sank. I knew this would be a devastating blow for her. It wasn't totally unexpected, because it was something Sue and I had feared ever since her return to work. But the reality of it was painful. At times Shannon presented herself very well; and at other times she had significant communication difficulties. Still, I was shocked when she broke the news.

"What happened? "

"They need someone to do advanced CAD, and I'm just not good enough at it. I can do boards, inventory, ordering, and everything else, but I just can't do CAD well enough..."

Shannon was in her car in a parking lot and was 'flooding'. She didn't know what to do or where to turn. It was a major setback in her recovery, and only increased our trepidation about her ability to survive on her own. I knew then that her termination by Casablanca had probably ended her hopes of a career in interior design.

We talked for half an hour while I tried to calm her down and coach her back to some state of normalcy. In the conversation, I learned that she had spoken to one of the owners of the company the day before and had revealed her accident and brain injury. Was that the *real* reason she lost her job? We'll never know.

Sue and I were powerless to help her. We anguished over her misery and disappointment, and felt guilty that we might have made a serious mistake in judgment about her ability to cope with the ups and downs of normal living. In our haste to let her return to a normal life, had we compromised her recovery by throwing her into an impossible situation rather than enrolling her in professional therapy?

It was time for us to find out the answer to that question. We decided that we needed to initiate another round of visits to physicians and psychologists. Doing nothing was no longer an option. We prayed that it wasn't too late.

Our first step was a return visit to Dr. Bradburn. He happened to be gone for two weeks, so we scheduled Shannon to see his partner, Dr. Manju Kandula. Dr. Kandula was kind and attentive, and assured Shannon that deep depression is totally normal and part of the recovery process. She felt that in time Shannon would overcome it. This, however, didn't make Shannon feel any better. The next step was a visit to a Neuropsychologist for testing and counseling.

Dr. Alan Gladsden was an expert in neuropsychological assessment and IQ testing. His plan was to measure Shannon's mental agility and life skills, and provide coaching on how to improve her abilities, self-image and confidence level. Hopefully, the outcome would be a healthier attitude, better coping strategies, and a fresh outlook on life.

...another test... just what I need... and right before the 4th of July weekend! ...

I woke up on Thursday morning with that established in my mind. The IQ test was supposed to tell me just how well I could comprehend life, thoughts, objects, and words. I went to Dr. Gladsden's office ready to sit down at a desk, complete a written test, say thank you, and be on my way. To my surprise, that's not what happened. It turned out to be an interactive examination given in two separate sessions. I was very nervous.

I never liked tests in school anyway, and those were on a subject other than *me*! Session one was a brief question and answer period with Dr. Gladsden, followed by a computer memorization speed test. First, he asked me to explain what I remembered about the accident, how I felt day to day, what I liked or disliked, and why I was always upset. Then I sat down at the computer and had no idea what it was all about.

...I can work on a computer... I know computer programs... I can type... I know how to turn it off... what is this supposed to show? ...

As I sat down to take the test, it brought back many memories from college. There was nothing to it, right? The computer test only took five minutes, and its purpose was to analyze my concentration and my ability to quickly look at data, respond, and move on. I thought I did pretty well.

After lunch, I came back for session two. It was the big question and answer session that consisted of a long talk about my thoughts regarding the steps I was going through for recovery. The test produced both positive and negative feelings. During a series of varied processes, Dr. Gladsden showed me flash cards that I needed to identify, memorize, and coordinate into objects. He spoke of incidents that I needed to state a resolution for. He quizzed me on mathematical equations. I wasn't very good in math before the accident, and I didn't do very well in trying to answer them.

Our long talk helped me see that my reactions, responses, and actions were not abnormal. I could easily see that it took longer for me to understand situations than other people, but if I had patience, I felt that I could eventually understand things as well as anyone else. He also heard more of my thoughts about my fears and rejections than I had told my parents or family. After we finished our counseling session, he confidently told me that what he had seen was typical of many traumatic brain injury survivors.

I honestly felt much better about myself as I was leaving his office. Then, the test results arrived. Looking at them today, I know a piece of paper, flash cards or a computer speed test do not tell you the whole truth. Some people are more efficient at some aspects of life than others. No one is good at everything. I may have deficits in some areas where my friends or family members excel, but I also have some other areas where I think I am better. Still, I was very disappointed in the overall results. That day I wrote the following in my journal:

...Am I really stupid? I think partly because my impressions and expectations are higher than the 'norm'. I want to be and have always been the overachiever. I feel like I have to prove myself to everyone always. Looking at these numbers he calculated today, I actually do need to prove I am capable of doing what I am asked or needed to do. The overall percentage number states I am in the high normal

range, but that is due to the high creative percentage mixed with the low analytical percentage. I can color in a coloring book, but can't add the objects in the picture together...

As I think back on that summer, those several physician appointments helped me recover some perspective. I began to realize that all the stories I continued to be told about the accident were actually true. I had to fully accept the fact that my life had drastically changed and I needed to start a new one. I had to stop looking so intensely at the past as though my life now would be the same. That's when I decided that I would do my own research to gather information that would help me personally understand what had occurred nineteen months before... and why I had become the person I was.

After my consultations and testing with Doctors Kandula, Gladsden and Bradburn, I was determined to make something more of myself. I began gathering copies of all documents and medical records pertaining to the accident. It took several weeks, but I finally received everything I asked for. They filled up an entire box. I then spent several months reviewing the material, and did gain a better appreciation for the situation.

Perhaps my biggest disappointment was the 'official' results of the IQ test, which stated that I was 'moderately to severely impaired'. I was determined to overcome those deficits, and I knew it would take time.

A vital part of trying to understand the accident was meeting some of the physicians who had saved my life. While I didn't get to meet as many as I would have liked, I did meet Dr. Jenkins, the surgeon from the Gwinnett Medical Center, who coordinated my care. What do you say to someone who saved your life? I didn't really know, but I thought it was important to thank him and let him see that his effort made a difference.

During this time, I continued to work full time at the furniture store. My thoughts were elsewhere, but I was still an effective salesperson. Because it was difficult for me to travel back and forth from Georgia to Tennessee for additional therapy, my Mom and I did some research and found a psychotherapist in Atlanta. I didn't want to see him, but my parents insisted. I really didn't have any choice... but I didn't have to like it.

I was uncomfortable with my new therapist from the moment he walked into the room. It seemed to me that he was goofier than me. Before my first visit, I wrote this in my journal:

...I am tired of doctors, but I have this feeling that this one will be the last one I have to see regarding the accident and the after-effects...

I was right. I was initially scheduled for eight to twelve weekly visits, but actually only saw him six times. He asked me many of the same questions that Dr. Gladsden had asked. I was bored. He also asked me about my involvement with activities outside of work like the church, IIDA, sports, friends, and school. I wanted him to be able to help me, but I just never warmed up to him.

I was worried about the thought of seeing and consulting another doctor. I hoped this new psychologist would help me to accept life as it was, and know everything that I was going through wasn't isolated to me. I didn't want more sympathy. I wanted to learn more about the situation, know why I was reacting the way I was, and I wanted to move on in my life instead of dwelling on the past.

I felt like I was ready to move on, and wondered why no one else was. It's apparent now that I was fooling myself. There was still much more to be done before I could lead a healthy, normal life. But it was also clear to me that more doctor visits weren't the answer. Besides, I was looking forward to a much more fun adventure with my Dad.

Whether or not she realized it, her consultations with various physicians and psychologists were a necessary and useful vehicle for Shannon's recovery. I am convinced, however, that the setting of a concrete personal goal and ultimate achievement of that goal was more beneficial to her.

The previous year I had hiked with Kelley and six Clinic friends from rim to rim in the Grand Canyon. Shannon had desperately wanted to go, but just wasn't physically up to it. I promised her that I would repeat the trek with her when I felt she was strong enough to endure the rigors of the trail. We had decided in July that we would go at the end of September.

During the summer, in between work and doctor visits, Shannon trained for our hike. Once again, it seemed to me that her best chance to chalk up a real success was through a physical challenge. We spent six days together in Arizona, talking about her life, her future, and her lack of direction. But it was the grueling hike down the South Rim of the Canyon; the hardships of the terrain in the Canyon; and the arduous walk back up to the eight thousand foot summit of the North Rim that provided the best therapy. For a few days, at least, Shannon was at peace with herself. She had proven that she could still compete physically, and it helped her self-esteem immensely.

It may have been wishful thinking, but I felt that she had now turned the corner. I knew there were still many highs and lows to come, but I was sure she was headed in the right direction.

...sometimes people accomplish things that make them feel better. After hiking through the Grand Canyon, I can say the word 'better' doesn't begin to describe how I feel. It's

been such a long time since I felt anything I had accomplished was really good. I do things here and there, and I continually suggest things to co-workers, but to have the right to say I walked thirty-three miles in two days carrying a thirty-five pound backpack through the Grand Canyon is an experience I am proud to brag about. I wasn't worried about me because I had trained for eight weeks before I went to Arizona, but I was worried about Dad. Yes, he has always been athletic and a part of whatever physical activity he could, but could he do this trek carrying a forty pound backpack for all those miles and worry about me at the same time? As we hiked past the 'finish line' today, I felt that Dad and I had bonded, acted and reacted again as we had done in my past life. It was a great feeling...

I had only been back to Atlanta for a few minutes, and as I walked calmly to my car, I almost felt like a real person again. Inspiration had hit me. I knew that I *needed* to really take control of my life again, so I immediately began evaluating where I was, what I was doing, what I thought, and how I was acting... and why. It was also time to get on with life.

I began to be more social. My football friends called me to watch, attend, or talk about games. I became more active with my Sunday School class, and particularly enjoyed practicing drama scenes for the children's Christmas festivities. I was promoted to manager once again at the furniture store. Customers were asking my opinion about layouts and designs for their home and work environments. I had my own apartment that I decorated in my style. I was in great physical shape again. My head was clear. But, for some reason, I had a strangely empty feeling. Things just didn't seem right.

Although I was staying busy and was involved with various people, I still felt alone. Football is only a sport. I would have appreciated the guys calling me for other reasons, too. Retail work was not that exciting. I was tired of sales. Even though I had been told that I did a great job,

I had much higher aspirations than being the 'sales queen'. After a great deal of thought, I determined that it was, once again, time for a change. My journal entry from December 12, 1997 reflects what was in my mind as I contemplated my future:

> ...what if I head back to Mom and Dad's house in Murfreesboro? I'm guessing the only way to know the answer to that will be to call home and ask. I have no idea what they will say to me. I begged to leave last year. What if they say no? ...

---TWELVE---

The Boomerang

Sunday, December 14, 1997, 7:30 p.m.

"Honey, Shannon's on the telephone... why don't you pick up the extension."

We talked to Shannon regularly on the telephone, but it was typically during the day. She would call me at work or Sue at home, so a nighttime call to both of us was reason for me to suspect that something was up. She seemed in good spirits, so I anticipated something positive... I just didn't know what.

"Daddy, can I come home?"

"Sure. We'll be here."

"I don't mean for a visit. I want to move back home..."

It took me about one-tenth of a second to react.

"I'll be there tomorrow with the truck..."

I knew she had to give a notice at work and would have to take care of the details of her lease for the apartment, but I wanted her to know that she would be welcomed home with open arms. As she talked I was thinking:

...in spite of the positive face she's putting on it, she still has problems that need to be addressed... it will be much easier for all of us if she's at home... here we go again... but it's for the best...

Shannon worked out a notice period with the furniture company and spent the New Year Holiday with friends in South Carolina. In the middle of January we reversed the moving process of seventeen months prior. This time it was from Marietta to Murfreesboro. While we were certainly happy to have her home where we could better support her, we knew we would again have to manage her frustrations on a daily basis. And we did.

Shannon's plan was to find a job, save money, move into her own apartment, and make friends. Unfortunately, she grew impatient, unfocused, and highly frustrated because things didn't happen fast enough to suit her. A note from her journal captures the essence of her feelings at the time:

...Dad and I took a long walk and fully discussed my perception of myself. He also gave me his fatherly advice on family, giving, job potential, moving on, and satisfaction with life in general. After two hours of conversation so in depth, I realized that 'I am never supposed to know my purpose'. My main job is to take life day by day. Life will never be exactly how I expect it to be and I can't count on things always falling into place...

The most difficult aspect of having Shannon back home was the aura that was created in the household. Everything centered on *her* needs, feelings and aspirations. It seemed that we talked with her constantly about setting realistic goals, the process of looking for jobs, how to present herself, how to prepare for an interview, and the value of patience. Her recorded thoughts at that time show just how difficult it was to make headway:

...I can't believe we're having this conversation again. I know what I want. I just don't think anyone will give me a chance. I am not stupid. I have this strong feeling that Mom and Dad don't think I can do it. If I am told how I am supposed to act another time, I will show them the worst way to act. Why can't I act natural? Am I a robot that someone can program to do what they need, not what I need? It makes me so angry. I am not who I used to be. Why try to act a way I don't vividly remember? ...

There was always a fine line between regulating her perspective while not undermining her self-esteem, and making her understand her capabilities and limitations. One wrong step inevitably led to alienation. Her perceptions of people, places and things were clearly out of kilter. Again, her journal recordings are insightful:

...I am worried about the way the people see me, especially my interviewers. My hair has grown back. No one can see any scars. I know what needs to be said. What worries me is the way I ask a simple question or explain an idea. I don't realize how confusing and misguided my words are until after I've said them. I know what I am trying to say. Why won't it come out that way? Half the time, I wish I could erase it and say it again... the right way...

During this time, I visited Dr. Bradburn several times to discuss my observations, and asked his advice about how to proceed. He reminded me that her brain injury was in the left frontal lobe, which controlled both perception and problem-solving abilities. While she could organize things, she just couldn't seem to coordinate her thoughts well enough to remember or sequence abstract ideas. Consequently, she took lots of actions, but they were not controlled or effective. In short, she spun her wheels quite a bit.

Dr. Bradburn also reminded us that it was approaching three years since the accident, and that in all likelihood Shannon's healing was complete. She was who she was, and any remaining deficits would probably remain for life. That meant her skewed perceptions, difficulty in phrasing sentences, emotional dependence, and mediocre problem-solving capabilities were here to stay. Our task was to try to help her be all she could be within the range of her resources.

While I had mixed feelings about moving back home with my parents, I thought I was fine mentally. I just needed a change to get life started in the right direction. I was convinced that the problem wasn't me, but the people I was dealing with. From my journal:

...Dad told me that a head trauma victim is typically healed after three years. I was fine after three months... I

can't believe that no one believes me when I tell them I am fine... *so what* if a few doctors had to screw my head back into place, a good car always needs a tune up, doesn't it? ...

I spent almost two months looking for a job, mostly in some clerical capacity. I registered and was credentialed at two staffing services, I interviewed for several positions at Middle Tennessee State University, and the Regional Office of State Farm Insurance. I thought the interviews went well enough, but my typing speed was too slow to qualify me for those jobs. The rejection made me angry and I wondered if anyone would ever give me a chance.

I got desperate after a few weeks of failure, and answered an ad for a design associate at Sprintz Furniture in Nashville. They were very nice and actually offered me a position. They said that I would start in a sales position and could slowly move into a designer position. Sales was old news to me and the current designers had no plans to leave anytime soon, so I put this job at the bottom of my list. Yes, I wanted to do what I studied and excelled at in school, but I just didn't want to return to sales. A February journal entry:

...Well, this month has had mostly lows. Now that I am thinking back, no good memories jump up... I am living free, but have nothing to show for it. Here is a perfect case of taking, not giving...

The first half of March was no better. The following passage from my journal tells it all:

...I am totally frustrated that I am still unemployed and no offers are remotely coming my way. I have no purpose and I don't want to be around. Why am I here anyway? This no job and no money thing is driving me insane. When I get over my self-pity, I am determined to have a job. I thought 'coming home' would be the best aid in confidence, savings, income, prosperity, and improved social life. We'll see. Slowly but surely I am feeling better about myself, but staying at home all day long is growing old. I might as well have stayed at the furniture store. At this point, considering that I have a comfortable living situation, I eat decently, and I have free time to play and investigate, why are my thoughts irrational and uncomfortable? ... but you know what... *welcome to life!* ...

My big break came on St. Patrick's Day. Kelley called to ask if I would be interested in a temporary position with GTE. I said okay. I needed something. Five minutes later, she called again to tell me to call the temporary agency handling the job, and suddenly I was employed. I was a little bothered about the GTE position because it was a temporary one, and because of the distance to travel. Enough of that... it was my lucky day, and I was finally getting started again.

I was both excited and nervous to be going to work. Excited because it gave me a sense of self-worth again; and nervous because it was in Kelley's workplace in an industry that I had no knowledge or experience. I was still very disoriented, even though I didn't realize how much until I look back at my journal notes a couple of weeks after I took the job:

...Now that I have been here for two weeks, I have discovered that I am not as smart or fast as I had been. Banging my head made me lose that. My newest plan is to work very efficiently and move up somehow. I need to move as soon as possible. I am very unhappy... living with Mom and Dad, working in my sister's work environment, not having extra money to spend, and no social life continues to take its toll on me as long as I think about it... I have also learned that time does lead to new realizations...

In my mind, April of 1998 was the turning point in my brain injury recovery. I was doing pretty well at my job, I was making friends, and I began to feel like a real person again. I knew I was different from other people in some ways, but I still thought I could be useful and productive. Somehow, with the help of my parents and co-workers, I was able to see that I was never going to be

171

successful if I was always self-centered, paranoid, and continued to act like a retard.

A friend at work kept telling me that I was okay, and that I shouldn't be concerned with what other people thought of me. I was who I was, and people could either accept me or not. He and I talked a great deal, and it greatly helped my perspective. It's funny that he said many of the same things as Mom and Dad, but coming from someone who didn't know me well, it just sounded different. My journal reflected my change in attitude:

...I think I am finally adjusting to this life. I still look forward to a life and place of my own. My workload isn't difficult. I spend too much time on certain projects and try to organize my manager's files, books, and spreadsheets, but I always complete my assignments. Frequently, I finish my work so quickly that I have time to research, learn, create, and update company databases. That surprises me. I think I am responsible and so does the company... Slowly, very slowly, I am becoming a part of the clan that knows each other and works together so much. I can be a part of a group. I understand that these people were Kelley's friends first, but they are spending time with me to know me better, not because we are related. That makes me feel wanted again. I thought I had a goofy, off-the-wall personality at times, but after talking to some of my co-workers, I know mine is not so lame...

Sometime in the spring of 1998, Sue and I noticed subtle changes in Shannon's behavior. She came home from work and talked about things she was doing, people she worked with, and plans for the future. We saw less brooding and complaining, and more anticipation. More importantly, we saw signs of improved concentration and focus.

Shannon was now beginning to think about looking for a permanent job and an apartment closer to where she worked. While we didn't discourage her, we reminded her that she would need to be settled and essentially independent financially before undertaking that step again.

Our plan was to pay off her car and continue paying for her college loans until she was able to resume responsibility for them, but we wanted her to be able to fund her apartment and other living expenses. She agreed, and it provided a meaningful goal for her to work toward in the next several months.

It is important to stress that Shannon didn't just change overnight. Her perceptive abilities seemed to improve slowly, but she still struggled with her communication skills and the mechanics of problem solving, and remained much too emotionally dependent on us. We also continued to coach her on dealing with her bouts of 'flooding'.

Sue and I worried about her being able to complete tasks on a computer while answering telephone calls, juggling commands from a boss and requests from engineers, and handle office politics. We feared a repeat of her experience at Casablanca Design, and fretted about what another disappointment like that would do to her. Strangely enough, Shannon never even considered the possibility that she might not perform at an acceptable level... even with her deficits.

For now, however, things were on an even keel. Shannon was holding a job, getting along with people, and was in a work environment where she had her sister for support in the event of a crisis. Then the unexpected happened again. This time, it seemed like good news; but it still took us by surprise.

---THIRTEEN---

The Hastening

Thursday, June 18, 1998, 2:30 p.m.

It seemed like a pretty ordinary day at work. My manager was out of town at a tower installation, and I revised, copied and sent a proposal to the parties involved; I assisted several of the technicians with their newest project plans... and fought with the ancient copy machine. Little did I know that this weekly battle would lead to a major change in my life. Fairy tales couldn't end up any better. What makes this really interesting is that it was totally unexpected. Here is what I wrote in my journal that very morning before coming to work:

...I am just still clueless about my abilities and what might happen... but everything seems to be so much better these days than two months ago... I won't even try to think or go back a year... but for some reason, I am still confused at which way to head... I need to find a motivation and a goal to go after besides get a new job... remember to stay focused on the idea that I won't find things easily...

I had opened every door on the copier in an effort to resolve the paper jam. No luck. As was typical, a waiting line was quickly forming and the jokes were flying. Mike threw out one of his popular 'Kehoisms'... basically, a really stupid pun or play on words. Most of them were massively absurd. I always tried to throw something back at him, but today nothing came to mind. I was too drawn to Mike's eyes scanning the fingers on my left hand. Somehow I knew that a friendship was about to be born.

We had seen each other around the office for the past few months, but really hadn't taken the time to talk very much. As fate would have it, we found ourselves on the elevator together that evening as we left to go home. I made a comment to him and we talked briefly as we left the building. It all started as innocently as that. That night

I wrote the following in my journal:

...I've lived through such a variety of changes... what could this one do? ...

I felt like I had a friend in Nashville now. Most of us were housed in small 6' x 8' cubes, and all of a sudden mine became the target for every stray rubber band he could find... which I dutifully returned periodically. We worked in a high-rise building near Centennial Park in the West End section of town, and I often got out to walk in the park during lunch. Soon, Mike and I began walking together on a daily basis.

I openly talked with my new acquaintance. I found him to be a good listener. He listened to my sob stories as well as the good memories I hadn't forgotten. I liked him, but I still wasn't sure how he really felt. A note from my journal during that period captures my thoughts:

... he has helped me in a lot of ways... listening, confidence, liking myself. It seems like a game though. It's interesting that I feel this easy and comfortable with someone I work with and have just begun talking to...

Mike's perspective:

I never saw Shannon as a recovering brain injury patient. Perhaps it's because I was too naive to look beyond her positive characteristics. But for whatever reason, I honestly just didn't think that much about it. Maybe that's the very nature of a head injury; what is so very traumatic to the patient and family is so totally invisible to the rest of the world. Those who didn't live through it simply don't know they are supposed to fret about it.

Shannon began working in my office during the spring of 1998, replacing another assistant in a cube across a hall from my own. After the brief, bewildering introduction that everyone has when they first start work, it took a week or two before I really said much to her. To some who are unfamiliar with office politics, that may seem to be a long time to make acquaintances with someone so close; but I couldn't let it seem that I, the single guy, was pouncing on the new girl. Rather, it was best to maintain an air of total indifference than to suffer the consequences that too much attention would inevitably ignite.

Ed, an older, very personable engineer who sat next to my cube, broke ranks first. As a friend, he naturally reported back to me with the results of his inquiry.

"Well, what's she like?" I quizzed.

Ed glanced to Shannon's cube then back to me. "She is the best listener I've ever met," he replied thoughtfully. That seemed to me a very unusual statement to make of one's first impressions. Clearly, Shannon was someone I needed to meet.

After a few weeks, we gradually became office friends. Fresh off of a failed 'on again, off again' relationship, I had no desire to date anyone for months, and *certainly* not someone from the same office. Still, I found Shannon charming and friendly, and it was hard not to stop by her cube occasionally throughout the day.

I also found that her playful nature complimented mine quite well. Seated at my cube, I would lob rubber bands over my cube wall, across the hall, and into Shannon's cube. My accuracy was measured with a quiet "missed me" to the very rare "dead on."

Every few days, she would gather all the projectiles from her bookshelf, her small potted ivy, and her hair and return them to me. Too polite *or* mature to fire the bands in return, she opted to simply hand them back to me with a half smile. I found that quite endearing.

Always concerned with her weight, Shannon declined to pack or buy a lunch. From years of experience, I can state with absolute certainty that the only way to lose weight is through maintaining a high metabolism, something that cannot happen if you skip meals and starve yourself. Shannon, however, was convinced that I was wrong.

Actually, she didn't need to lose any weight; she just thought about it all the time. So I started sharing my cafeteria lunch; splitting it two-thirds for me and one-third for her. I would place her portion on a paper plate and deliver it to her cube with the simple command, "eat." She would always resist, but never to the point where I thought the attention was unwelcome. She actually lost three pounds in the next month.

After a few weeks of this ritual, lunch evolved into *our time*. It was now August, and when the weather was mild we would take strolls though the Park and the 1920's bungalow neighborhood that adjoined our office. Inspired by the classic architecture and fine gardens, Shannon discussed in confidence her years in design school, her years and accomplishments competing in gymnastics, and of the accident that changed everything.

Convinced of the depth of her handicap, she often dwelled on her mental and emotional shortcomings, and how she was now different than the outgoing leader she was before. There was no doubt that she had been through a lot, but I couldn't get past the notion of *SO WHAT?* I didn't know her before the accident, so all I could judge her on was the way she was now... attractive, fun, and inspirational. From what I could see, all she needed was her self-confidence and everything would be perfect.

As the summer grew, so did our friendship. Eventually, we thought of dating, but this was hindered by her living with her parents fifty miles away. Considering her past, late evenings on the town were not an option. Instead, we opted for weekend activities such as hiking in a nearby park, renting canoes and picnicking down by the lake. It was a beautiful summer, not unlike one you might imagine Sheriff Andy Taylor having in Mayberry.

We would drive around the city, pointing out and discussing the history of unique architectural details, a hobby we both had in common.

"That's classic Georgian over there, isn't it?" I would ask.

"What? Look at the roof," she would correct, "that's Regency."

And so it went... the typical stuff any young couple talks about, right? No matter, we enjoyed our time together. More importantly, Shannon seemed more at peace with herself and the world around her.

As summer progressed, Sue and I noticed that Shannon seemed a little less edgy and somewhat more content. When she first moved back from Georgia, she was absolutely obsessed with keeping up with all of her old friends, as though moving on would be disloyal to her past. Now that she had social interests in Tennessee, her obsession eased palpably.

She complained less to us, and didn't seem at all bothered when we were out of town for a week or so. We wondered what was happening. One night at dinner, we found out.

"Mom, I made a new friend at work. His name is Mike Kehoe, and he's a communications engineer."

Sue and I glanced at each other with that 'ah ha' look on our faces.

"So, tell us about him," I asked.

"Oh, he's been with GTE for about five years or so."

"Is he from Nashville?"

"No. He's from New York."

"New York?" Sue again looked at me.

"Where in New York?" she asked.

"Skaneateles. It's in the Finger Lakes Region near Syracuse."

We learned that he was thirty-four years old and the youngest of three children; was a good listener, had a sense of humor, staunch values, liked the outdoors... and absolutely didn't care about her brain injury.

His father was a Chemistry professor and his mother was in an administrative position with a local vocational school. They lived in a tidy bungalow on thirteen well-maintained acres, lived modestly, and had a strong work ethic and love of the environment.

For the first time in three years, Shannon was enthusiastic, and we could see that he had played a role. We were watching her personality and sense of self-worth re-emerge right before our very eyes. This wasn't supposed to happen, was it? Brain injury survivors gain all their improvement in the first six months or a year. Maybe so... *but not in this case!* Indeed, it was turning into a pretty good summer.

Mike again:

Eventually, it was time to meet her parents. By this time, I already knew that Shannon came from a very close and decent family, something we thankfully had in common. I was not at all nervous on the evening I was invited to dinner at their house. Partially, this was due to the fact that at age thirty-four, not much makes you nervous; but more importantly, I genuinely wanted to meet her parents myself.

Following Shannon's directions, I found myself looking down their long driveway to the large house and manicured lawn, and remembered Shannon's only advice:

"Just don't drive on the grass." Fearing an accidental dip of a wheel off the unfamiliar pavement or, Heaven forbid, a drip of oil from my aging Nissan onto the white concrete, I briefly considered parking on the street. I shook it off and parked in the circular drive near the front door. I thought:

...what am I getting myself into? ...

I don't remember much of the evening except that I had a wonderful time. I couldn't have felt more welcome. Even Haley, the family dog, who was famous for guarding the family, took to me warmly. *Really.* I'm not saying that just because my in-laws will read this. The evening went just as well as I knew that it would. It was then that I thought Shannon and I had a future.

Later, when we wanted to spend more time together or perhaps get an early start to the day for a long hike, I would be invited to spend the night at their house. I slept in Brian's room, across the hall from Shannon's. After long evenings following dinner, reviewing family photo albums of Shannon, and *watching more college sports than I had seen in my entire collective years prior*, I would retire to the bedroom and sleep extremely well. One morning, after I was more comfortable, my mischievous side got the best of me.

Sometimes, staying across the hall from your girlfriend tempts you into doing some particularly stupid things. I mean to say she's right there, across the hall. Just two doors away! That's like twenty-five feet, much better than the fifty miles I was accustomed to. And my weird sense of humor prevailed. I should have known that I was destined for a rather embarrassing event.

Yep. I'm talking about that one fateful morning when her mother turned into the hall and caught me; and I gasp to think of it to this day, crawling into Shannon's room... *on all fours*, dressed with my socks and shoes on my hands proclaiming to Shannon that something terrible had gone wrong and I needed her help.

Caught in the act I was. Of course, her mother got quite a laugh out of it. Heaven knows what she thinks of me to this day. Nonetheless, I didn't get thrown out. Now I was pretty sure things were going to be okay.

We found Mike to be smart, engaging, and a bit off-center. *A perfect match for Shannon.* She smiled more, communicated better, 'flooded' less, and seemed more confident. Whatever his motivations, Mike had been just the therapy Shannon needed. All of a sudden, she was more aware of the world around her, and started thinking of how she fit in.

Shannon's nose was essentially obliterated in the accident, and while the cartilage was still intact, it was distinctly crooked and would someday need to be repaired. She had lost her sense of smell, and we thought surgery might correct both the cosmetic and olfactory problems. Up to now, however, she had shown absolutely no interest in having another surgery. Her appearance was again becoming more important to her, and she decided it was time for a 'nose job'.

What was most gratifying to us was the initiative Shannon took... *and the maturity she displayed*, in inquiring about surgeons, evaluating insurance coverage, scheduling appointments, and assessing her options. Six months before, she could neither have understood all the details involved nor been emotionally independent enough to make the decision to proceed.

All of a sudden, in the fall of 1998, a new, stronger Shannon was emerging. Instead of the self-centered, immature pessimist we had seen for the past three years, we were seeing a more confident, positive, and reasonable young adult. We were astonished at the transformation that was taking place... and Dr. Bradburn was confounded. In his experience, it was a rare occurrence.

We didn't know how much more improvement Shannon might make, but she now clearly qualified as a traumatic brain injury success story… and we were very grateful. We were curious to see how she would handle the impending surgery and it's aftermath. Once again, Shannon was in for another test of strength, will, and mental acuity. Would this be a triumph or tragedy?

---FOURTEEN---

The Partnership

Monday, September 21, 1998, 7:05 a.m.

I arrived at Centennial Hospital in Nashville early, and was immediately taken back to the pre-operative room and started on medicine and the dreaded IV. The TV entertainment while prepping for surgery was a tape of President Clinton's testimony about the Monica Lewinsky affair. *By then I was ready to be knocked out.* After an hour, the nurse came in, gave me my last pill and rolled me away to surgery. I said goodbye to Mom and zonk, I was out cold.

Here is what I wrote in my journal early that morning before going to the hospital:

...Today is another day that will be with me forever. I am really glad this weekend was so good. I needed it to prepare me for this week. Mike and I went hiking at Stone Door in McMinnville. Sadly enough, I was happy the heat and length of walk didn't bother me, but it did Mike... I slept decently, but have this very uneasy feeling. Here is a positive note: needs to be done for medical and cosmetic reasons. Picturing it scares the hell out of me. Thinking of each process gives me the willies. I think what gets me the most is the fact that I know what is happening rather than just being here. The last time I was in the hospital they didn't know if I would make it through the day...

Sue and I were greatly relieved as Shannon was wheeled back into Room 402. Dr. Orcutt had assured us that everything would be fine, but we openly worried about how the anesthesia might affect her brain function. Our apprehension was unfounded. While Shannon was groggy, she was fully aware of her surroundings, and even displayed a refreshing sense of humor. Now it was just a matter of healing time.

Nurses are always concerned about patients' urinating after surgery, and their constant prodding produced one of those quips that made us feel much better.

"Shannon, we need for you to try to go to the bathroom."

"Okay," Shannon responded half-heartedly. "Since I have this nice flowing gown with the back end open, I guess all I have to do is back up!"

We all had a good laugh.

Kelley arrived early in the afternoon and looked mortified at the sight of Shannon's bandages. It took her back three years to a very unpleasant time that she would just as soon have forgotten. Shannon reassured her that she was fine, and Kelley seemed relieved. Mike came in a little later and brought some levity to the proceedings with a steady stream of 'Kehoeisms' on hospital food, beds and lousy patients.

The next morning couldn't come quickly enough to suit Shannon. She was tired of being watched and monitored... and for once, was actually hungry. She and Sue couldn't get out of there and home soon enough.

On Thursday of that week I wrote the following. I think it pretty well sums up my feelings about the surgery and how I felt about myself:

... Believe it or not, my face was only a little bruised and swollen and I didn't care. I had family and my new friend there to tell me they loved me no matter what. Now I am anxious to take my splint off. One week until I see my honker. I know I am not a model or close to one, but they have problems too. Right? Today, I feel so much better about myself. I can't really explain why. I don't understand myself. Maybe it is Mike. He is an outsider that puts up with

me and listens to me about anything and everything... One thing I especially like Mike for now is that I have more on my mind than myself. I have been stuck on me for three years. How self-centered is that? ...

Recovery from the surgery went very well. I puttered around at home, and in no time I was able to get the splints out of my nose. It was really nice to be able to breathe freely again. My nose looked a lot better, but I still had no sense of smell. That continues to this day. I also had lots of time to think. The following entry from my journal summarizes my thoughts two weeks after the surgery:

...I for some reason have a different perspective on my life, where it needs to go, the thought processes, emotions, work, just about everything... The week went well and I seem to be fine, Mike came down both days. I am a mess of emotions. I am not really sure what has gotten into me. My brain is on a roller coaster. I will say that one well-known saying continues coming back to me when I am alone thinking of the day, the time, experiences and situations I have been through: *patience is a virtue...*

I was extremely restless for the next couple of months. I don't attribute that to my brain injury though, because I've always been someone who likes action. I was bored at work, and except for Mike and Kelley, I had no reason to be there. I liked the people, but I wanted to do more and I knew there was little chance of moving up. It was then that I decided to begin looking for a permanent job again. Here are some snippets of my thoughts during October:

...I still have no idea what I am all about. I used to think talking or writing 'cured' me, but these days I am not so sure. I write and talk so much that it confuses me, much less what anyone else thinks... I am amazed at how well Mike and I get along. It just clicked as soon as we became friends. I feel I tell too many things to Mike as it is. I wonder if my talking so much is an asset or downfall... I don't know where my drive is. I seem to have my ideas and mind in too many places, concerning so many different topics. I understand that focusing on a few topics at once is fine, but I am lost in which topics to begin focusing on. He listens to me. Now, whether it goes in one ear and out the other is a good question. I talk to Mom and Dad, but I have done that my whole life. Do they still listen to me or just let me blow off steam? ...

After recovering from the surgery, my outlook was definitely better, but I still missed my friends and I missed being social. I also missed having my own home. Mike would have none of my brooding, however, and did his best to get my mind off the past and on to the future. One of his cures was a Halloween Party at the end of the month.

I had never really celebrated Halloween. To me, the dressing up part was great, but celebrating death, destruction and terror never thrilled me. Another co-worker and new friend invited Mike and me to a party at one of the Nashville clubs. Since it was on short notice, we had to scramble around to find costumes.

I had no interest in using my old costumes... especially the hospital scrubs and lab coat. Mike was determined to be something loony, which describes his personality pretty well. I eventually found a French maid uniform, and he created a Dilbert costume, which really isn't a stretch of the imagination if you know Michael at all! Let's say that night was interesting... Dilbert and his French maid, or as Mike called it, Dilbert on the 'Mother of all Dates'. It was really good to be free again.

We were happy that Shannon now had someone outside the family with whom she could share her feelings. Her spirits were noticeably higher, but as all parents, we worried about her fragile psyche in the event that the relationship waned later on. Still, things were much more normal, and our conversations seemed more on an adult level. Whatever was going on between Mike and Shannon, it had a positive effect on her recovery. We hoped it continued.

As winter approached, we began to sense that Shannon was restless again, and her comments led us to believe that she was ready for a new job and a place of her own. Her confidence was returning and she was more rational most of the time now. Accordingly, we felt better about her ability to live independently, particularly since she would only be a short distance away.

While she said she liked living at home okay, having a job and a friend in another city just wouldn't work for much longer. The long drive to Nashville was creating early mornings, and spending time with Mike after work led to late evenings. She was simply wearing out physically.

She was convinced that she could make it on her own financially if she could find a permanent job with a stable income, so she began a job search in early November. Once again she had a goal...*and once again,* she went after it with gusto. It pleased us immensely to see the potential of the new Shannon.

Strangely enough, I was excited about the challenge of a new job because I had more confidence than I had previously. That was due to Mike's influence. He made me feel that I was worth something again, and it filled me with energy. Anyway, after all this time, I thought I was finally finding myself. I just needed to follow through, show patience, be honest with myself, see reality not fantasy, and move on day by day with some progress toward success.

Part of my reality check was a review of what I had written in the past year or so in my journal. One day out of the blue, it hit me! I noticed that I constantly jumped from story to story and feeling to feeling. *It dawned on me that my writing mirrored my train of thought,* and probably reflected the way I was coming across in interviews. I vowed to be more focused in my upcoming interviews, and concentrate on how I communicated with potential employers. *It worked.* My journal entry for November 18, 1998 says it all:

...I got a job! I got a job! Can you tell I am excited? I am excited, but must remain under control with confidence, glow, and stamina. The best part about this position is that it deals partly with what I learned in graduate school. It is creative. It is imaginative. It is people oriented and it is not the regular behind the desk type of job. I am the Advertising Coordinator for a local real estate company... At this moment, it would take a lot to crush this feeling. Ultimately, a company is willing to let me do what I am confident of... Wait until I tell Mike. Why is he the first person I want to tell? I feel like I have known him for years not months. Coming from me, I shouldn't be surprised... I have a full-time job with benefits much needed...

The next few months were active and productive. First, I was invited to spend Thanksgiving with Mike's family at his sister's house in Cincinnati. I was worried about creating a good impression, but it worked out fine, and I really enjoyed getting to know them. After that, we went to art exhibits; shows at the Tennessee Performing Arts Center; we went hiking and canoeing; occasional sporting events; had dinners at nice restaurants; and we redecorated Mike's house. I really felt alive again.

I still had moods I couldn't control, but Mike never let them bother him. He had a sixth sense, and knew when to give me space and when to give me support. Nonetheless, there were now many more *ups* than *downs*. A note from my journal in last days of 1998 pretty much sums up my perspective at that time:

...It is the end of another year. What did I do this year? Let's see: move to Tennessee, start a new job, then

another new job, make new friends through my work environment, learn to work professionally in a business, and find the man I want to spend the rest of my life with. Overall, it might be considered a positive year. I know that in January I was lost and still looking for a path. In '98, I had researched my medical records and realized something serious had happened, but it never occurred to me that I wouldn't have 'recovered' until several years had passed. I look back now and wonder why I was so convinced that nothing was wrong with me. The next big question will be how I see this situation five, ten, twenty years after it happened...

Mike's view:

When I first became aware of Shannon, it was clear that she had much more potential than she believed. It was easy to see that she suffered from bouts of discouragement and lack of faith, no doubt from losing her dream of being a designer. She was adrift in the business world when all she wanted was a fair chance to prove to herself and the world that she was a capable person.

I knew exactly what she felt like. I, myself, grew up shy and with a great lack of confidence, never really seeing how I fit into the overall puzzle. I was unforgiving of my own shortcomings, and didn't feel that I measured up to others who seemed so comfortable with themselves. Naturally, not too many people found this attractive, so I found myself alone much of the time. 'It's got to be me' was my rationalization.

However, my perspective was altered by a change of environment and several supportive friends. These friends didn't judge me; they actually seemed to like me for who I was. I gradually found adventure and confidence through long bicycle tours through the Mohawk River Valley, mountain climbing, and kayaking. I found my place, and I belonged. Shannon deserved the same chance that I had been given.

For so many years Shannon had built her life around the expectation of becoming a leading designer, but with that dream stolen, she felt lost. She constantly complained that her drive was gone, her memory was gone, and she just didn't know who she was anymore.

There had to be something wrong with her, right? Well, I'm sorry, but I wouldn't have any of that. Her memory? It was better than mine, for goodness sake. Anyone would feel bad if they really knew how forgetful they could be. And yes, perhaps the accident had changed her, but doesn't life change everyone? Just not in the same way. That's the very reason we're all unique.

I thought that if I could give Shannon some exposure to design, I could rekindle the drive in her. I invited her to my house for some consultation. Although I felt that I had done a fairly acceptable job of decorating, most walls were still painted a generic 'builder's white', and useful items such as tools and sports equipment were left conveniently in the open.

Unable to fund a large make-over, we compromised with a few gallons of paint, a little trim work, and some inexpensive measures such as putting all my stuff in a place called 'away'. I was sure that I'd be forever poking though boxes to find my Walkman, but after a few weeks, my humble abode was transformed into something that closely resembled a comfortable home. I was most impressed.

The New Year began very well. I was getting comfortable with my job, and found a nice apartment closer to Nashville. Here is what I wrote in my journal near the end of February:

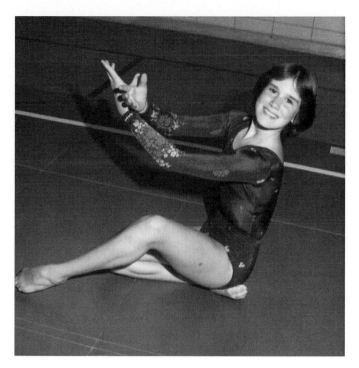

Shannon in gymnastics... Age 10.

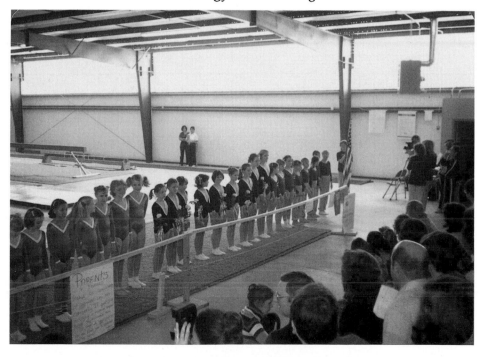

Budding gymnasts at Club Meet... 1982.

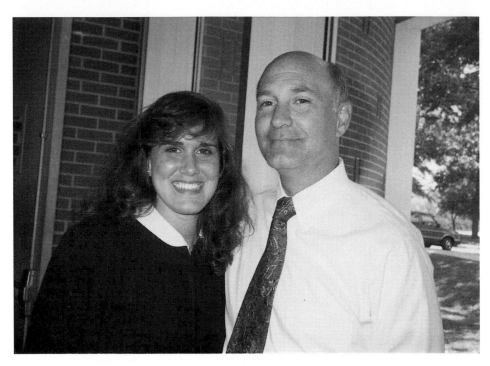

Shannon and Don at her UGA graduation... 1993.

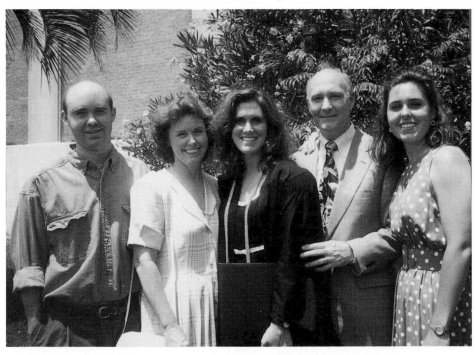

Brian, Sue, Shannon, Don & Kelley at
Savannah College of Art & Design graduation... 1995.

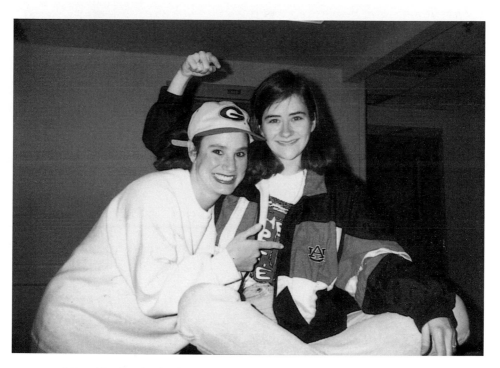

Kim (Sothen) Black and Jennifer (Beaulieu) Beherns... 1995.

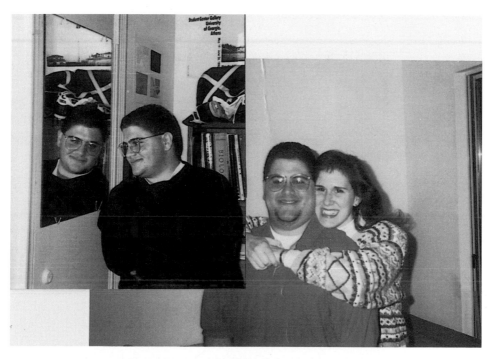

Samy Iskandar and Shannon at UGA... 1992.

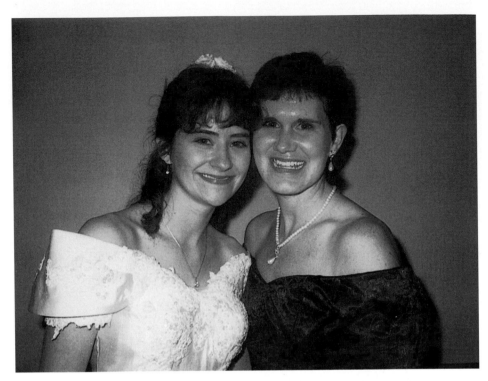

Jennifer and Shannon at Jenn's Wedding… May, 1996.

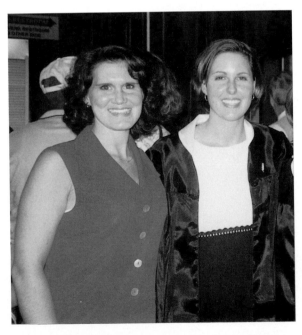

**Shannon with her sister at Kelley's graduation
from Middle Tennessee State University… May, 1997.**

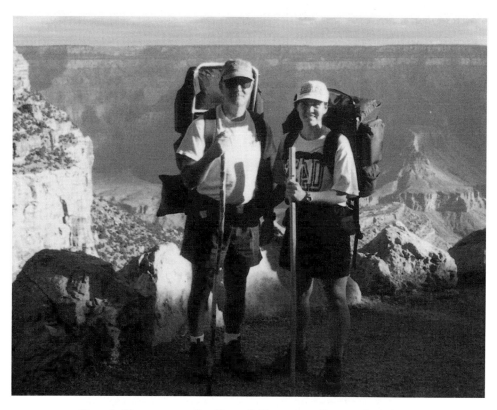

Don & Shannon at the Grand Canyon... September, 1997.

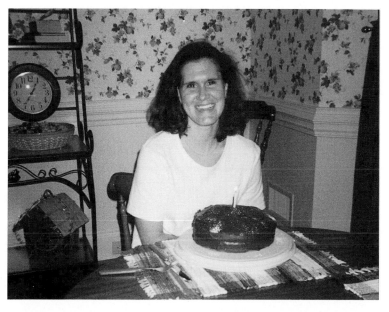

Shannon on her twenty-seventh birthday... August 26, 1998.

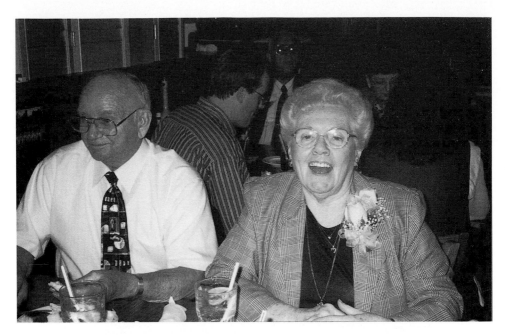

Shannon's Grandparents... Claud & Mary Catherine Eason... 1999.

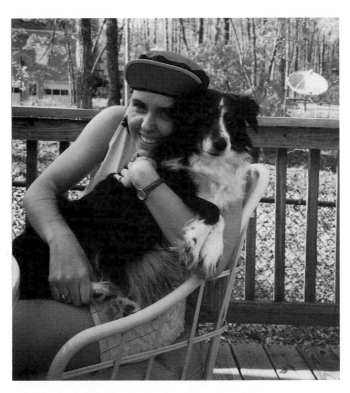

Kelley and her best friend, Haley...

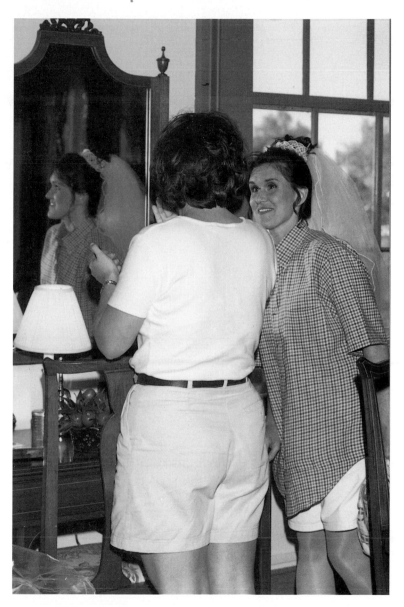

Kelley & Shannon preparing for the Wedding...

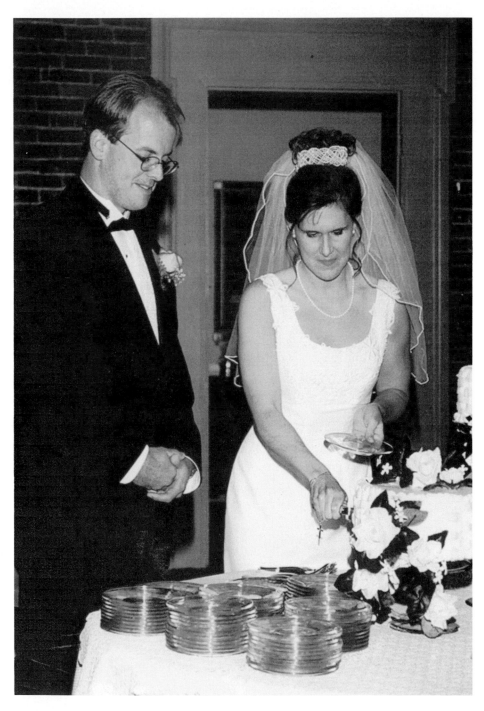

Mr. and Mrs. Michael J. Kehoe at the Reception…
September 25, 1999

...This year started off on a high note – I have my own home, I live closer to the man I deeply care about, I have a steady job, I am drawing, revising, and hopefully correcting Mike's house plans (utilizing my degree), and now headed to Mississippi to meet one of his best friends... Robert Mitchell is a very interesting person. He has a personality that you could never say no to. Now I understand why Mike is such good friends with him. Mike is fun, but Robert is so outgoing and spontaneous, he pulls Mike slightly out of his conservative shell...

As a matter of fact, I was beginning to *feel* like a new person. Another entry in my journal summarizes my thoughts as spring approached:

...What else can we do this month? I am still amazed that my concentration, my perspective, and my emotions are 50% more focused today than a month ago. I honestly believe that creating trail adventures, attending theatrical and musical performances, and traveling around the state with Mike contribute to this shift in my personality. My thoughts are on something other than medicine and Shannon. I like this. And the fact that I have someone to spend time with, share experiences with, want to become closer to, and who likes me for who I am now, not who I used to be... My self-perspective is better. Okay, that may not be a word, but it looks good to me... I know for a fact that one main reason for accepting myself is Mike. He means the world to me. I'm not sure how I got so lucky. It isn't my place to question that...

While I liked the duties of my job with the real estate company, the demands of the job were too much. I struggled to keep up with the vast amount of work and the outdated equipment I was using. At first, I thought it must be me, but I soon found out that there had been several other individuals who had the same problems, and had subsequently left the position.

I wasn't anxious to change jobs again, but I knew that I also couldn't keep up the pace forever. I was frustrated, but not like I had been in the past. I was dealing pretty well with the disappointment because so many other things were going well, and because Mike and I were able to find time to enjoy the outdoors regularly. Working hard physically has always had a therapeutic effect, and all the backpacking, hiking and camping helped me keep a positive outlook.

We are now in an age where more women like to hit the trail and get dirty. I am one of them. I like the challenge. Experienced or not, rough terrain or not, every trip is different. In April, Mike and I decided to test each other on a camping trip to Fall Creek Falls State Park in Middle Tennessee.

We plodded up and down the paths through a calm, peaceful, and preserved woodland. The backpacks were a little too heavy because we didn't pack as efficiently as the experts recommend. Mike continuously told me that he wanted to take everything to be on the safe side. That's where we didn't fully agree, but he hadn't hiked or camped in a long time so I let the old saying 'live and learn' prove its meaning.

The hike was demanding, but enjoyable. We had beautiful views of the waterfall while hiking out of the canyon, and often stopped at a quiet overlook to look over the deep glen. During those times, nothing seemed more comfortable and relaxing to me... just nature and a happy couple.

The very next weekend, we decided to spend a little more time with nature. But this time, it took place at Cheekwood, the Tennessee Botanical Gardens located in Nashville. For me, it instantaneously became a wonderful place to look at natural beauty and inspire creativity. Not much time had passed when I discovered the view and inspiration had also hit Mike. But I'll leave the story to him.

❖❖❖

Mike's story:

The hike at Fall Creek Falls was strenuous, but to say the least, the view of the waterfall and the forest was spell binding. At one point, we sat on a large, flat rock on the edge of the overlook and soaked it in. After some time had passed, Shannon began to rise, and I said, "sit a while longer." The trip proved to me what I already knew. I loved her; we made excellent companionship, and could overcome anything together. Looking at the falls, I could see the past, but looking at Shannon I could see the future. The moment was magic and just then, without planning to, I thought about asking a question.

"I... I..." Just then, a noisy group was making its way down to the overlook and, unfortunately, the moment was lost.

"Better get going," I said, as I slowly stood up, helping Shannon with her pack.

Shannon looked at me, but didn't say anything. I think she knew what I didn't say. I felt... well, I don't know what I felt. Expectant and sad, all mixed together. I thought of the advice my friend Robert had given me only a few weeks earlier:

"She's a good woman. You're going to marry her. Why wait?"

The next weekend we joined Cheekwood, Tennessee's botanical gardens, art museum and school, located less than a mile from my house. It was mid April, and the spring flowers were in full bloom. I thought Shannon and I could both draw some inspiration from the gardens, and possibly join an art class in oil painting. Well, *I found inspiration all right.*

It was a beautiful, crisp morning as we walked up the path from the drive to the main mansion. Surrounded by a rich profusion of flowers and ornamental shrubs, I stopped adjacent to a small stream and shared the one good idea of my life.

"Let's get married," I said.

"OK, sure; lets do," she answered, as if I was joking.

"I'm not kidding. Lets get married. Will you marry me?" I asked again.

Her dark eyes stared at me with amazement as she answered a few second later.

"Yes!" she exclaimed, as she jumped into my arms. Oil painting would have to wait.

Ring... ring... ring...

"Hello."

"Hi Dad... it's Shannon."

"Hi honey. How are you doing?"

"Fine. Can you get Mom on the other telephone?"

"Sure. What's up?"

"Mike and I want to talk to you two."

Well... I wasn't certain, but I thought I knew what was coming. Sure enough, I was right. They excitedly told us of their plans to get married.

"Michael... are you sure you know what you're getting yourself into?" I teased.

"*I think so,*" he responded. "To tell you the truth, I just can't imagine living the rest of my life without Shannon."

So there it was. Shannon had found a soul mate, and one of her major worries in life was going away. It was as simple as that. Mike had ignited something in Shannon that no physician, psychologist, therapist or family member could. A zest for life and a purpose. After three and half years, Shannon was really back in the mainstream.

The next few months were the happiest times we had experienced in quite awhile. Sue and Shannon worked on details of the wedding, which was planned for the end of September. Because the two of them were so organized and detailed, no stone was left unturned. As a result of their efforts, I had no doubt it would be a tasteful, beautifully choreographed event.

Shannon and Mike continued to canoe, hike, camp, and visit friends and relatives. They attended Shannon's ten-year high school reunion in Birmingham in June, and went to Skaneateles, New York to visit Mike's parents in July. Shannon also decided to once again look for a job that would complement their lifestyle.

Through it all, Shannon handled the whirlwind calmly and with greater maturity than we thought possible. She still had some communication, concentration, and decision-making deficits, but her perspective and confidence level had improved markedly, and she began working around them just as though they were simple logistics problems. All in all, her transformation in the last twelve months had been nothing short of remarkable.

Shannon's moment:

September 25, 1999 was a glorious day. I started the morning with the following entry in my journal:

...Today I will begin a new life. And to make these changes, I am not even the slightest bit nervous. I feel so confident that this is right and very meaningful that I must be breaking a rule somewhere... Since the time we first met, many changes and experiences have happened, yet it never altered our thoughts or how we focus on life. From my understanding, that means the relationship is honest and everlasting...

As Kelley and I parked at the Governor's Club main house, I couldn't say anything except that everything was perfect. The weather was great, the house stunning, the landscape, flowers and floral arrangements were beautiful, and the atmosphere was elegant and cheerful. It was true, the ceremony wasn't going to take place in a traditional church, but utilizing this outstanding, historical home was unique.

…Here I am in the dressing room. What am I thinking about? Resolutions, in case I make a mistake or forget what I want to say to Dad or Mike. Okay, nobody will know if I mess up or not, but still, I'll know. Jennifer, Kelley and Mom are here to get dressed and to help improve my looks. I am not actually concerned about looking flawless. Mike has told me several times that he makes joking comments about models or celebrities, but I am just as good-looking as they are…

Knock… knock… someone was at the door.

…I need to go now. I'll write more tomorrow on the plane… are you ready? …

It was Dad. He came in and we talked briefly before we started down the stairs for the ceremony. I know he was still very uncomfortable after his back surgery at the end of July, but he really seemed pleased for me. We were both pretty emotional.

At the last minute, I wondered how I looked, or if I would say things correctly… mostly the traditional nervous, jittery wedding feelings hit me. Well, the time had come. As Dad and I walked out, I asked myself, "Is this for real? Am I doing this?" Right then, I caught Mike's eye and had no doubt it was one of the best decisions I had ever made.

The wedding was truly an affair of the heart… and soul… and mind. The ceremony went pretty well, and I only half lost it while trying to talk to Dad. He kissed my cheek, told me everything was fine and sat down. Mike and I exchanged vows and then it was official… Mr. and Mrs. Michael J. Kehoe.

During the reception, Reverend Muse asked me about the necklace I had wrapped around my wrist. I explained that it had been a Cross that my grandmother had left for her first great granddaughter, and that it had been given to me while I was recovering from my accident.

While she wasn't physically present for this memorable day, I felt a small part of her was because I was wearing her Cross.

Mike's moment:

Our wedding day was just as magical for me... the groom.   Like Shannon, I didn't feel nervous at all.   My family had flown in a day or two in advance, and I had been plenty busy with picking them up at the airport and making arrangements to get everyone to the rehearsal dinner.

Robert, my groomsman, and his wife Angela were staying at my house; everyone else was at a hotel a few miles down the road.   I have a hard enough time keeping my own life arranged, but since we didn't lose anybody, I guess we had to call it a success.

I should have been tired because I had only slept for an hour or two the previous night.   Actually, I was so filled with anticipation that I really felt rather good.   As the day unfolded, however, I did begin to worry that I was forgetting something.   I do that when I'm tired.   Did I have Shannon's bags for the honeymoon loaded in the car?   Did I have the airline tickets?   Does my brother, Danny, have the marriage license and rings?   I finally collected myself and decided that we were all set.

I wondered where Shannon was. Was she excited? I sat upstairs in my appointed room for about an hour, mostly by myself.   I could hear family entering below and my nieces melodically banging on the grand piano.   I had been warned to stay upstairs and away from the windows, lest I see Shannon too soon. I dutifully complied.

As Robert was with his wife, and my brother fashionably late as ever, I was alone with my thoughts... feeling oddly left out of the events unfolding below:

...my goodness, is this where I'm going to get married? ... really much too nice for us... since Shannon and her Mom made most of the arrangements, I really haven't had a chance to walk around the mansion.. a fine job renovating the house... furnished with antiques... very nice... we're surrounded by million dollar homes in Nashville's most exclusive gated golf community... it looks like a million dollar wedding... it isn't, but let them think what they will... I'm just happy to be getting married outdoors, where I feel a comfortable bond between God and nature... I'm glad we avoided the strict formalities that are not part of our lives... an outdoor wedding seems perfectly appropriate for us...

After getting dressed in our tuxedos, Robert looked out the 'forbidden' window and caught a glance of Shannon outside in her gown.

"Mike," he said with his characteristic Texas accent, *"You've done real good.* Shannon is absolutely beautiful."

I was ecstatic. Now I started feeling a little jittery. Soon a new life would begin.

A three-piece string ensemble, fresh off of a tour in Ireland, provided the music. As both our families are mostly of Irish decent, we had requested classical music with a blend of traditional Irish melodies. Standing by the gazebo, I focused on the strings to calm my racing nerves. I scanned the small gathering for family and friends, and tried to look composed. In reality, I think I was smiling like a loon.

The strings slid into the richly beautiful melody of Pachelbel's *Canon in D* as Kelley and Jennifer emerged from the house, and slowly marched down the isle.

...this is it! ...

Then Shannon walked from the house, escorted by her Dad. I was swelled with emotion...*she was stunning*. She looked at me, smiling, and I practically choked with happiness. After a short pause, they proceeded up the isle. I could see Shannon trying to hold in her emotions. I, too, fought back the tears.

The wedding was like a dream... I floated though it much as water floats in a river, largely unaware of what was happening around me. At one point I heard the vows that Shannon and I had written together, but that's about it. Then Shannon paused to address her Dad. As he gave me her hand, Shannon wished to thank him for all the love, support and patience that he has unselfishly offered through the years, and especially through her recovery.

"Dad... I..." was all she could say before breaking down into tears.

"I know, honey... *I know*," he reassured, hugging her. Everyone knows of the special bond between the two, and there wasn't a dry eye in the crowd.

Before I knew it, the ceremony was over. *We were now married*! Everything seemed perfectly natural because this was how my life was intended to be.

Throughout our courtship, Shannon told me many times how much I helped her restore her life. I'm glad, certainly, but she'll never know how much she helped me in return. In her, I have found both a soul mate and best friend... *and life has never seemed better.*

---FIFTEEN---

The New Shannon

Editors Note: This chapter has only been minimally edited so the reader can get a better feel for Shannon's everyday use of words and phraseology. She, of course, wanted everything corrected, but we thought it would be more instructive to leave as much as possible in its original form.

I suppose at some point in our lives, everyone asks, *"Who am I?"*

What's interesting about that question is that you don't see what you're *not* looking for. You have to look deeper for that. Unlike a lot of 'normal' people, when I ask, "Who am I?" it's because I really want to know. But for me, it wasn't that simple. I just couldn't remember.

Through pictures and journals, I pieced together my life as it was before the accident. *This isn't me*, I thought. *Here is a girl who burns the candle at both ends, 24-7. An overachiever, determined and confident.* I was determined to be a leading designer; managing my own firm by the time I reached thirty. My name would be known in high society. I was going to be *somebody*, and would prove that I was better than everybody else. I was on my way.

Whoever that was, that's not me today. I don't want to be like that anymore. I never lost my drive, but it is clear that my definition of success has now changed. I no longer have to prove myself to everyone. I'm not better than everyone else; I think I'm just average. But that's okay, I like who I am. Too bad it took a hit on the head to knock some sense into me.

By looking at me today, you would never know that I came so close to dying. While telling people my story, they find it hard to believe. It's even hard for me to believe sometimes. At first appearances, you don't see any outward damage. I still have all my fingers and toes, and can move around fluently. However, upon closer inspection, I carry scars.

Depending on my hairstyle, you might notice one scar that extends like a headband from ear to ear. Or, at the beach, you can easily see the ten inch abdominal scar that extends from my breastbone down to 'where the sun don't shine', closely complimented with dimples from the GI tube and catheter. In the words of my doctor, "*Ooh! That's a doosy!*"

Thankfully, I don't have any scars on my face. The plastic surgeon did a wonderful job rebuilding my face to a very close resemblance of its original state. No one knows that much of my face is formed from titanium. Only my immediate family notices a slight difference. For one, my eyes are now set back further, and my cheekbones are not quite as high as they once were; all of this created from my high school senior picture. Why couldn't they have just given the doctor a picture of Julia Roberts instead?

Despite the success of my facial reconstruction, I have permanent nerve damage that has partially numbed my upper lip and destroyed my sense of smell. In the beginning, my numbed lip made speech a little difficult and drinking from a glass messy, but fortunately now, I've adjusted to this. More dramatic though, was the loss of smell, a common ailment of people with similar facial injuries.

Initially, it bothered me that I could no longer enjoy the smell of bread baking, dinner cooking, or even fresh cut flowers. I used to worry that I couldn't smell smoke or tell if gas was leaking. But now, I have grown accustomed to this. Except for the fear of an undetected fire, I honestly don't think about it.

Subtler yet, just as having a cold, with my loss of smell came a loss of taste. I can taste sweet, sour, and bitter, but otherwise food can be rather bland...*except chocolate.* No woman can ever forget how good chocolate can be!

After recognizing all of the other injuries, my broken hip was the least of the doctors' worries, and alone received little attention. But what can you do, you can't cast a hip, can you? By and large my hip has healed, except that it can no longer endure the stress of jogging, something that was once a very big part of my life. After only a mile, my hip will throb with pain, and I must stop. Today, to stay in shape, I do the best I can by walking and jogging through all of the imaginary terrain on the treadmill, but I'll never again enter a road race. Not as a runner.

Soon after we began dating, Mike bought a bicycle for me so I could ride along with him. I knew riding was a major part of his life, and was thrilled that he wanted to share this experience with me. The last time I had ridden a bike, it had one speed and you pedaled backwards to stop. This new bike, however, came with fourteen speeds and two brake levers, whose operation I couldn't quite grasp. I was frustrated and felt like quite an idiot for having so much difficulty with something children take for granted.

But what really upset me was how easily I became excessively breathless when riding up even the slightest hill. My body needed oxygen that I just couldn't provide. As a result of the accident, I have a marked decrease in aerobic capacity that continues to this day. For this reason, I have learned to compensate with workouts of lower intensity.

Still, there was no hiding my limitation on the bike. Mike suggested walking up the hills we encountered. *What would people think?* I didn't want to look weak and helpless, and my ego was hurt. Not wanting to disappoint Michael, I grew resentful of the bike, and gave it up for good.

These days, I feel that my lungs are fine, just not as strong as they had been previously. I've accepted that I will never be the athlete that I was, but that doesn't stop me from being as active as I can. I may have been forced into early retirement, but I don't dwell on it anymore.

The physical ailments have been easy to overcome. The challenges I face with brain trauma, however, are not that simple. By bruising my brain tissue, I had to re-program myself. This assignment required a combination of processes including reasoning, perception, sensibility and intellect to complete. These senses are the foundations of who we are. Stability and understanding of these are necessary to balance emotions and communicate clearly. Let me tell you how nerve racking this is.

As you know, a great amount of my neurons have been misplaced or destroyed, so the connections that form reason and memory struggle to connect. The best way to explain this recovery is trying to make order out of chaos. I've come a long way from seeing giant bunnies eating trees in the front yard or believing that all cable installers are evil... *but I'm still not so sure about that last one.*

Perception can be in the eye of the beholder. Is the glass half full or half empty? By definition, perception has several meanings; something conceived in the mind, an abstract or generic idea generalized from particular instances, and the quality or state of being aware... *especially of something within oneself.* Many times, how I perceive a situation contradicts the truth, and that can be a problem.

Do you know how many times in the past few years people have told me, "That's not what I'm saying; you've got that wrong"; or "that's not what we meant." To me, perception is not so much how I see the world, but how the world sees me. Do I look as though I know what I am doing or am I struggling? Are they questioning me? Did she complete the assignment quick enough? Does it contain all the material needed? Is she confident enough to show us what she has done? Her desk is so neat and clean, does she actually work or just tidy up the space?

It seems to me that I still have a little trouble with this perception thing. A simple question from Mike such as, "Honey, have you seen my binoculars?" might be interpreted as an accusation that I had misplaced them rather than Mike simply saving some search time. Naturally, I become defensive and snap back. A prime example of making a mountain of a molehill.

When this happens, it makes perfect sense that Dr. Bradburn jokingly reminded me that sometimes his real job was in construction rather than medicine. His responsibility was to help me build an easy access highway rather than a spaghetti junction.

Today, I am relieved to have regained much more control over my emotions, but unfortunately not quite all. For the most part, I have full control of my feelings, but I'm still prone to lose it with little warning. Little things that typically never bothered me can now set me off. It is an impulse reaction. For example, while I listen to the American Anthem before a sporting event, I become teary-eyed. I have no idea why I want to cry. Or when I wait in line for movie tickets, I get angry because I purposely let someone else jump in line first... another instantaneous reaction.

True, I've never been as calm as my brother over situations, but at least I could think my way through them instead of just reacting to them. My first reaction is usually an immediate response of anger or sadness rather than looking at the whole picture. I may or may not ever have the ability to overcome these emotions, but I am learning to handle them.

Another impairment is the continual struggle with communicating. That road is still under construction and more than likely won't ever reach completion. When I am involved in a deep discussion, casual or business, my thoughts fly in every direction. My concentration is lost.

The challenge of processing too many stimuli at one

time is a constant battle. Basically, during these discussions, I follow the line of conversation and I know the answers to the questions asked. I *could* have the perfect answer to them, but my answers are so lengthy and far from the truth that it seems I am just mumbling ideas out loud. The words I verbalize aren't the words I genuinely mean to say. I realize I've made this mistake after everyone looks at me with a confused look on his or her face. That's when I say, "So you *ARE* paying attention," to make it funny and to cover up my blunder.

Few people I work with know of the accident and impairments, so mistakes such as these are not looked down upon. I don't consciously associate the word confusion with the accident. As days, months and years pass, I have basically forgotten about what had changed my life. I have become accustomed to my deficits. Really, I wish I could report that all is rosy and I am fully recovered from my trauma, but I'm not. I will never fully be.

What is important in life? We must recognize that each of us has limited time alive. Enjoy this time; use it before you lose it. Every day is a bonus. I say this because I look at things differently. You don't always need to *be* the best at whatever you try. You just need to *do* the best you can.

My perspective on life is different. I still have wants and desires, but not as extreme as before. I recognize things as they are... not how I wish they would be. I'm glad to be able to wake up in the morning and see the rain, sun, flowers or whatever.

I understand that how I see things isn't always right. Nobody's perfect or always right. But I'm willing to accept that now, when I couldn't before the accident. I expected perfection... *from myself and everyone else*. Imperfection was more than a little annoying to me. I've now learned that to survive in life, you just have to accept it and move on. I don't think about it anymore.

The grass is greener on the other side, right? But is it really? Too often, we want to be in someone else's shoes... more money, bigger house, fancier car, or whatever. I don't do that anymore. I'm thankful to be me and have what I have now. I've learned that everyone has problems, and being in their shoes only means exchanging one set of problems for another.

There is so much pressure on people today. Society says that you must look good, be young, be thin, *and be cool*... and if you don't see yourself that way, you're a failure. If you go by the magazines or what you see on television, then you are letting someone or something else create who you are. I don't feel that pressure anymore. I am who I am, and I live my own life. Eleanor Roosevelt had some good words of advice on that subject:

"Believe in yourself. You gain strength, courage, and confidence by every experience in which you stop to look fear in the face. You must do that which you think you cannot do."

I've learned some other things about life, too.

First, you must set limits on your mind and your body in order to function completely. You can't live on the edge and expect to be effective. If you do, sooner or later you'll pay for it. You don't have to give up everything; you just need to slow down.

Second, remember to make notes, take pictures, and make scrapbooks. They remind you of who you are, what you've done, and what your life has been about. *That is life*!

Third, life is full of obstacles, but you must go ahead and live your life in spite of problems or troubles. How boring would life be if there was no pain anyway?

Fourth, without the support, love, and strength I received from my friends and especially family, I wouldn't be where I am today. When you give a little, you get a lot.

Fifth, I can't think as quickly or clearly as other people, but after reviewing my journals for the past five years, I am convinced that I continue to improve each day.

I've learned to take the time to listen, interpret, and decide exactly what is happening before I respond. It helps a lot.

Well, in a nutshell... *who am I now?* I'd like to think that when people see me, they see a kind, considerate person with *some* smarts. I live every day basically just as everyone else does; I keep up-to-date with current events, I handle household chores, I go to work. Overall, I think I'm a normal person, and I'm content with this.

What I've learned during my recovery is to value the life I have, and every moment that we have to share with each other. *So don't blow it!*

---SIXTEEN---

The Unpredictable Brain Injury

There is no doubt that Shannon is a brain injury success story. You can clearly see, however, that it doesn't mean her brain functions as efficiently as it did before the accident.

We must remember that thousands of the pathways her brain used to absorb, interpret, process, and act on information were eliminated at the moment her head impacted the windshield of the automobile. These pathways can never be re-established. In their place, her brain has constructed new avenues to accept and transmit information. The problem is that they are simply not as proficient as the old ones. In basic terms, sections of the superhighway have been closed, and she is now forced to use some back roads to get to her destination.

We must also keep in mind that her reduced brain efficiency is partially due to blood vessels and tissue in the frontal and temporal lobes of her brain being permanently destroyed, altering the performance of these portions of the brain. As a result, many functions performed in these areas have been compromised and can never be restored to their original capacity.

Again, the concept is easier to visualize if we use a common example. We can clearly understand that if she had cut off the tips of a couple of fingers, she would still be able to use the hand, but not with the same dexterity as before. This is what happened to Shannon; we just can't see the extent of the damage inside her head.

At the risk of being redundant, it should be re-emphasized that every brain injury is unique, whether it is a mild concussion from a fall off a bicycle, a stroke, or a severe closed head injury resulting from an automobile accident. And while there are some common elements of brain injuries, standard courses of treatment, and predictable stages of recovery, it is critical that every case be treated individually.

The patient's age, general health, socio-economic background, religious and cultural beliefs, and family support are just as vital to recovery as structured rehabilitation programs and therapy. It was our experience that *the* most critical factor in Shannon's recovery was family participation in the entire process... from the immediate treatment when she was unconscious to the long-term therapy decisions. There is no substitute for knowing the patient intimately. This allows for a more focused approach to treatment and rehabilitation.

If you are ever thrust into the position of caring for a brain injured friend or family member, what should you expect? First you must understand that the consequences of traumatic brain injury may be cognitive, physical or emotional... or a combination. Below is a very nice summary that I replicated from the Web site of the Brain Injury Association:

Cognitive consequences can include:

- Short term memory loss; long term memory loss.

- Slowed ability to process information.

- Trouble concentrating or paying attention for periods of time.

- Difficulty keeping up with a conversation; other communication difficulties such as word finding problems.

- Spatial disorientation.

- Organizational problems and impaired judgment.

- Unable to do more than one thing at a time.

Physical consequences can include:

- Seizures of all types.

- Muscle spasticity.

- Double vision or low vision, even blindness.

- Loss of smell or taste.

- Speech impairments such as slow or slurred speech.

- Headaches or migraines.

- Fatigue, increased need for sleep; balance problems.

- Pain.

Emotional consequences can include:

- A lack of initiating activities, or once started, difficulty in completing tasks without reminders.

- Increased anxiety.

- Depression and mood swings.

- Denial of deficits.

- Impulsive behavior.

- More easily agitated.

- Egocentric behaviors; difficulty seeing how behaviors can affect others.

From reading the story, you can easily see that Shannon experienced most of these disorders for at least some period of time. She was fortunate that most of them were only temporary, but a few of these disabilities do still remain. She has just learned how to live with them.

We did not intend this book to be a comprehensive or authoritative brain injury reference. We'll leave that to the experts in the field. What we did intend was to share the story of one family's battle with a largely hidden, but extremely widespread problem in today's world.

Had Shannon chosen not to drive on that fateful night, our struggle could have been avoided. We can't change that now; and as a result, we will be living with the consequences of that choice forever. We want our story to be a warning to parents, teens, and young adults that one seemingly harmless lapse in judgment *can* be very debilitating or fatal. Accordingly, we encourage families to talk about lifestyles and choices.

We also hope that our saga provides some comfort to families of brain injury victims and the victims themselves. We want you to know that you are not alone; you are not an aberration; and you are most definitely not without hope. The sad fact is that not everyone will recover enough capacity to live a relatively normal life... *but many will.*

While our story appears to have a happy ending... *does it really?* No one who knew Shannon before the accident will ever believe she is just as well off now as before her brain injury. The sad fact is... we'll always wonder how much she was compromised, and how much of her potential will never be realized. We'll just never know. But somehow it really doesn't matter to us... we love her just the way she is now!

Finally, we wanted to share some key observations and lessons we learned through the years as we dealt with Shannon's injury and rehabilitation:

- Brain injury victims don't readily accept their injury. They remain in denial for a long period of time.

- The victim and family unit will never be the same again. Each individual will have to make adjustments in lifestyle to accommodate for the long-terms effects of the injury. For example... Shannon can do many physical things, but she cannot share Mike's passion for bicycling. One fall on her head would be catastrophic.

- Family members will have intense feelings... and will feel guilty at times for having those feelings. Parents will ask why this happened and where they went wrong. Family members will also ask why they have to sacrifice because of someone else's indiscretion.

- Families of victims need a great deal of support and help. It is necessary to ask friends and neighbors for assistance... both in the early days and later when progress seems to be slow or non-existent.

- Families always want the old person back, but it is usually not possible. Families and friends must accept that this is a different person, with a different persona and needs.

- Use the victim's innate talents, hobbies and passions as tools in the rehabilitation process. In Shannon's case, physical conditioning, drawing, and her passion for University of Georgia athletics were vital to her recovery.

- Determination, tenacity and exercise are excellent fuel for recovery.

- The family must do all they can to coach the victim to concentrate on what they can do... not what they can't do.

- As frustrating as it may seem, there are random factors that may have more of an impact on recovery than *all* the most carefully planned therapies combined. In Shannon's case, it was Mike. The minute she quit focusing on herself she started to improve dramatically.

- *Normal* encompasses such a broad spectrum of personalities, talents, capabilities and behaviors that people who didn't know the victim before the injury might never see residual deficits because they have nothing with which to compare. Also, over time, even those who knew him or her will gradually accept the new person for who they are now.

Oh yes, there is one other meaningful piece of advice that we'd like to offer. The late Jim Valvano, former North Carolina State Basketball coach and broadcaster, was asked to speak at halftime of an NC State game while dying of cancer. He could hardly support his body as he trudged to center court. He gave a very inspirational message to players and fans, and as he finished, he summoned up all the energy he had, and bellowed to the crowd:

"Don't give up... don't ever give up!"

EPILOGUE

Saturday, March 3, 2001, 6:38 a.m. *Ring...ring...ring...*
"Hello."

"Mom, it's Shannon. My contractions are five minutes apart. I called Dr. Ellington and she said I should come to the hospital."

"Are you okay?"

"I'm fine. We're about to walk out the door. We should be at the hospital in twenty minutes or so."

"Well, just be careful. Dad and I are on our way."

Sue and I got out of bed, dressed, ate breakfast, and were out the door for our five-hour drive from Monroe, Georgia to Franklin, Tennessee. After concluding a twenty-six year career as a health care administrator, we had moved back to Georgia only a few months before so I could pursue a Doctorate in Political Science at the University of Georgia.

As we passed the spot of Shannon's accident, we glanced at each other with a psychic communication that's only possible after a thirty-four year marriage and many shared experiences. It seemed improbable and ironic that only 1938 days ago we passed this *very same spot* coming from the opposite direction at the end of our journey to the Gwinnett Medical Center. Now we were at the beginning of a journey to the Williamson Medical Center in Tennessee for the birth of our first grandchild.

"Last time we were headed toward what we thought was death... *today*, we're headed toward life," she said.

"It looks like we've literally completed the full circle, doesn't it?" I responded.

Tara Marie Kehoe was born at 10:13 a.m. Once again, the miracle of life had been bestowed upon us... and it was indeed a time to *smile and jump high*!

BIBLIOGRAPHY

The major references for this book came from journals kept by Shannon, Don, Sue and Kelley; personal recollections of other family members; and medical records from Gwinnett Medical Center, Middle Tennessee Medical Center, and NHC Health Center.

We also found some interesting and useful sites on the Internet that allowed us to fill in gaps in facts or understanding of the medical elements associated with traumatic brain injuries. We have listed these web sites below, and suggest that the reader visit some of them. They are educational, stimulating, and sometimes even disturbing.

Brain.Com: www.brain.com
Brain Injury Association, Inc: www.biausa.org
Brain Injury Information Page: www.tbilaw.com/home
Brain Injury Resource Center: www.headinjury.com
InteliHealth: www.InteliHealth.com
National Resource Center for Traumatic Brain Injury:
   www.neuro.pmr.mcv.edu
The Brain Museum: www.brainmuseum.org/index/htmlx
The Joseph Corpina Foundation: www.corpina.org/info.htm
The Voice Inside:
   www.geocities.com/Area51/Nebula/5443/index-psych_tbi.html
WebMD: www.my.webmd.com
xrefer...the Web's reference engine: www.xrefer.com/search

ABOUT THE AUTHOR

Donald J. Lloyd spent twenty-four years as a medical group executive before retiring in 1998. He is now President of The StarLight Group, a health care consulting company located in Monroe, Georgia; and is enrolled as a graduate student in Political Science at the University of Georgia.

Mr. Lloyd received his Bachelor of Business Administration Degree from the University of Georgia in 1967 and Master of Business Administration Degree from Georgia State University in 1974. He was awarded Fellow status in the American College of Medical Practice Executives in 1979.

During his career in medical administration, Mr. Lloyd was an active speaker on health care administration issues, managerial ethics, accountability, and health care policy. He has also written numerous articles on those same topics; and is the author of **HEALTHCARE 2010:** *A Journey to the Past,* and co-author of **TRIALS TO TRIUMPHS: Perspectives from Successful Healthcare Leaders.**

ABOUT THE AUTHOR

Shannon L. Kehoe is a wife and mother who lives in Nashville, Tennessee. She is also a traumatic brain injury survivor.

Mrs. Kehoe received her Bachelor of Arts Degree in Interior Design from the University of Georgia in 1993 and Master of Arts in Interior Design from the Savannah College of Art & Design in 1995. Her aspirations for a career as a designer were cut short by an automobile accident shortly after completion of her master's degree.

This book would not have been possible without Shannon's permission, and indeed, her active participation in the process. She has written in a journal almost daily since childhood, and it was her private thoughts, observations and feelings recorded in these journals that provided the most poignant and insightful entries in the manuscript.